THE
MICROWAVE

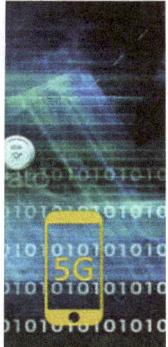

Are
dangering
).

The Diary of an Electrosensitive
Brian Stein CBE and Jonathan Mantle

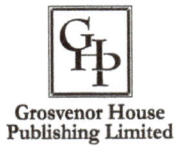

Grosvenor House
Publishing Limited

All rights reserved
Copyright © Brian Stein and Jonathan Mantle, 2020

The right of Brian Stein and Jonathan Mantle to be
identified as the author of this
work has been asserted in accordance with Section 78
of the Copyright, Designs and Patents Act 1988

The book cover is copyright to Brian Stein and Jonathan Mantle

This book is published by
Grosvenor House Publishing Ltd
Link House
140 The Broadway, Tolworth, Surrey, KT6 7HT.
www.grosvenorhousepublishing.co.uk

This book is sold subject to the conditions that it shall not, by way of
trade or otherwise, be lent, resold, hired out or otherwise circulated
without the author's or publisher's prior consent in any form of binding or
cover other than that in which it is published and
without a similar condition including this condition being imposed
on the subsequent purchaser.

A CIP record for this book
is available from the British Library

ISBN 978-1-83975-349-7

'We are taking advice from a small, self-appointed circle of insiders who reject all research showing harm, and who set safety limits.' **Brian Stein, UK**

'We are taking risks of the sort that no rational society on earth should take.' **Professor Martin Pall, Washington State University, USA.**

'We should have ethical permission for people who are going to be exposed to 5G. Thirteen persons make decisions for the whole world – as opposed to 250 persons who have signed the independent scientific declaration.' **Professor Lennart Hardell, Sweden.**

'The non-thermal effects on our cells, organs and tissues do damage at energy levels that may be hundreds or thousands of times lower than those that cause significant heating. Our governments and health authorities are doing nothing to protect us.' **Professor Andrew Goldsworthy, UK.**

'The car was not invented to be safe, it was invented to sell. Lots of people died. Only consumer pressure eventually forced car manufacturers to introduce seat belts. It's the same with mobile phones.' **Dr Andrew Tresidder, UK.**

Contents

	Pages
Introduction	xi
Significant Milestones	xiii
1 One of Us is Mad	1
2 A Brief History of the Diseases of Civilisation	7
3 Into the Electrostorm	73
4 Britons Enslav'd?	147
5 Doctor, Doctor	156
6 The Scientific Silence	167
7 Free Russia	174
8 Follow the Money	182
9 The Birds and the Bees	230
10 One of Us	243
Afterword	257
Chapter Notes	264
Glossary of Terms	270
Useful Websites for Research, Information and Advice	272
Useful Publications	273
Acknowledgements	275
Appendices and Links to Key Independent Scientific Studies	276
The Authors	279

This book is dedicated to all those who suffer from ES and are tortured by the advances in the roll-out of this technology.

Also to the brave scientists who are risking their funding and careers to expose the truth about the industry and industry bodies meant to protect our health.

'I have no doubt in my mind that at the present time, the greatest polluting element in the earth's environment is the proliferation of electromagnetic fields. I consider that to be far greater on a global scale, than warming, and the increase in chemical elements in the environment.'

– Dr Robert O. Becker, twice nominated for the Nobel Prize -

'Man conquered the Black Plague, but he has created new problems – EMF pollution.'

– Professor Yury Grigoriev, Russian Federation -

'The explosive recent increase in radio frequency radiation and high-frequency voltage transient sources, especially in urban areas from cell phones and towers, terrestrial antennas, Wi-Fi and Wi-Max systems, broadband Internet over power lines, and personal electronic equipment, suggest that like the twentieth century EMF epidemic, we may already have a twenty-first century epidemic of morbidity underway, caused by high frequency electromagnetic fields. The good news is that many of these MF diseases may be preventable by simple environmental manipulation, if society chooses to pay attention. Unless public outrage intervenes, I'm afraid that our 'diseases of civilisation' will only get worse. Good science alone is never enough to force sensible public policy. Only citizens can do that.'

– Dr Samuel Milham, USA

'The effects of non-ionizing radiation are the same as ionizing radiation in slow motion.'

– Professor Oleg Grigoriev, Russian Federation

Introduction by Brian Stein CBE

There are over a million severely Electrically Sensitive people around the world today.

They are generally ignored.

There are a quintillian – 1 followed by 18 noughts - more microwaves in our atmosphere today than naturally occurred 30 years ago.

This fact is generally ignored.

Every day of the year there is published peer-reviewed research showing that EMFs cause serious health issues.

This research is generally ignored in the UK. These health issues include cancer, dementia, behavioural problems, and brain tumours. Damage to the blood brain barrier, damage to the nervous system, damage to the unborn child and damage to the heart and fertility.

The million ES sufferers can all confirm that the EMF that they can feel causes all these health issues.

All these issues 'ARE' caused by ionising radiation and recognised as such, caused by thermal effects.

Research shows that exactly the same issues are caused by non-ionising radiation over a longer time scale, by biological effects.

The Governments of the world make significant revenues from the wireless industry and regularly sell off the EMF spectrum to the industry for billions of pounds.

One of the biggest advertisers in the media is the wireless industry. The largest donor to cancer research is the wireless industry.

Cancer Research UK does no research into EMF effects, yet regularly states that there is no evidence that microwaves cause cancer. Whenever there is publicity about EMFs causing cancer or health issues, the government, Public Health England and Cancer Research UK defend the industry, saying there is no research proving EMFs cause cancer or ill health.

The World Health Organisation has classified EMF as a 2B carcinogen 'possibly' causing cancer.

The media report that the 2B classification is the same as coffee, and therefore probably safe.

Some of the research is showing that EMFs might be as carcinogenic as tobacco.

The press regularly report the rise of cancer, but it is a mystery, or caused by diet, drink or drugs. No mention is made of EMFs.

The ES people would argue that many of the medical mysteries: sick building syndrome, ME, gulf war syndrome, and sudden death syndrome are caused by a combination of sensitivity to EMFs and chemicals. They are ignored.

The progress of these mysteries can be traced to the advancement of microwaves in our atmosphere.

Cancer, dementia and other diseases caused by EMFs are following the same trend.

This relationship is ignored.

Although the governments of the world are strictly controlling and battling the use of cigarettes, drink, poor diet and drugs the rise of cancer continues, as does the growth of EMFs in the atmosphere. There is significant growth in cancer and dementia in the young. Cancer is no longer simply a disease of old age.

Regular reports in the press highlight behavioural issues in children because of their use of computers and Wi-Fi. The scientific prospect is generally ignored that EMFs may also cause these issues, as research is confirming.

Research from France, Germany and Sweden is suggesting that low level microwave emissions (Wi-Fi) are more biologically active to animal cells than higher level emissions.

We are now bathing our children, pregnant women and unborn children in these emissions 24 hours a day.

We have not learned from the history of cigarettes, or asbestos that the authorities hid the truth from us to protect the economy.

Like the tragedies of child abuse by Jimmy Saville, and the disaster of Hillsborough, we will find that we have been lied to and the guilty have been protected by the media and the authorities, while the research necessary to prove their guilt was already there.

Significant Milestones

1972 Motorola in the USA enters the race with AT&T to develop the first portable 'wireless' telephone.

1973 Martin Cooper of Motorola makes the first mobile phone call.

1975 The American scientist **Allan Frey** reports that non-thermal microwaves such as those emitted by mobile phones can induce changes in the blood-brain barrier in white rats, the animals whose biology is closest to humans.

1981 1G is rolled out.

1983 The first commercially available mobile phones appear on the market without any government safety studies or checks.

1992 2G is rolled out. **David Reynard** brings the first American cancer and mobile phone-related lawsuit. Mobile phone stocks plummet. **ICNIRP** is formed as the industry-funded regulator.

1993 Tom Wheeler, president of the **Cellular Communications and Internet Association (CTIA)** in America commissions and funds epidemiologist and law graduate **George Carlo** to run an 'industry-friendly' Wireless Technology Reseach (WTR) programme.

1994 There are 90 million mobile phones worldwide.

1995 George Carlo starts work.

1996 The USA Telecommunications Act is passed. Om P. Gandhi loses his research funding.

1999 There are 200 million mobile phone users worldwide. George Carlo presents the WTR findings to American cell phone industry leaders and according to Carlo is escorted from the building. Tom Wheeler of the CTIA rubbishes Carlo and his findings.

2000 **The Stewart Report in the UK** advocates the 'Precautionary Principle' regarding the use of mobile phones. In Germany, mobile phone operator **T-Mobil** commissions the **Ecolog** study into the health dangers of mobile technology. The study finds unfavourably in terms of carcinogenic and genetic effects and is buried by T-Mobil.

2001 3G is rolled out. There are 500 million mobile phone users worldwide.

2003 Professor Leif Salford at the Rausing Institute in Sweden confirms the findings of Allan Frey and others.

2005 The IEEE in the USA further relaxes radiation safety thresholds on mobile phones. **Switzerland** issues a health warning to every citizen regarding the use of mobile phones and Wi-Fi.

2009 Business executive **Innocenzo Marcolini** wins a legal judgement against his employers citing protracted mobile phone use as the cause of his brain tumour. The Italian court bases its ruling on the independent research of **Professor Lennart Hardell**. Marcolini's employers appeal.

2011 4G is rolled out. 'Electrosmog' protests in Brussels.

2012 The Marcolini verdict is upheld in Italy, with the judge rejecting the ICNIRP industry standards in favour of the independent work of **Professor Lennart Hardell**.

Professor Yury Grigoriev's work in Russian on the health hazards of electromagnetic fields becomes available in English.

There are 1.9 billion mobile phone users worldwide.

2013 In the UK, with national debt running at £1.1 trillion, the UK Government auctions £3.5 billion worth of 4G wireless bandwidth to mobile phone companies such as Vodafone, Orange, O2 and T-Mobile.

The UK Health Protection Agency continues to insist that the **ICNIRP** safety thresholds are adequate and that electrosensitivity is a 'psychological' condition.

The President of Belgacom in Belgium tells children that mobile phones can be dangerous and bans Wi-Fi from the executive floor of his offices.

Settlements are made in favour of claimants suffering from mobile phone-induced health damage in **Israel** and **Australia**.

2014 There are 2.5 billion mobile phone users worldwide and over 50,000 microwave masts in Britain.

2015 190 scientists from thirty-nine nations submit an appeal to the UN and World Health Organisation for stronger protective exposure guidelines regarding microwave radiation and electromagnetic fields in the face of increasing evidence of health risk.

2016 The US government-sponsored National Toxicology Program releases the findings of its two-year study confirming the health risks of cancers caused by non-thermal wireless radiation from mobile phones. NTP leaders are accused by independent scientists of playing down the findings in the interests of 'big wireless'.

2018 In the United States, the independent scientific peer review of the **National Toxicology Program** concludes there is 'clear evidence' that radiation from mobile phones causes cancer.

In Britain, eighteen years on from Sir William Stewart's report, the **UK Health Protection Agency** continues to disregard the 'Precautionary Principle' with regard to wireless technology and the use of mobile phones.

236 independent scientists who have collectively conducted over 2,000 peer-reviewed studies worldwide, sign a petition calling for safety reviews of the wireless technology required to enable 5G and the **'Internet of Things'**.

2019 The largest ever studies undertaken by the **National Toxicology Program** in the US and the **Ramazzini Institute** in Italy conclude that low-level radio frequency exposure from masts and Wi-Fi and high-level radio frequency exposure in heavy mobile phone users show clear evidence of cancers.

NTP researchers in the US come under pressure from the US Government and 'Big Wireless' to distance themselves from their findings.

The Radiation Research Trust Conference 'Radiation Health 2019: Get the Facts' in London attracts leading independent scientists from around the world.

There are 5 billion mobile phones in the world.

In San Francisco, USA, the **'Phonegate'** class legal action is launched against mobile phone companies on the grounds of hazard to the health of children and pregnant women.

In Turin, Italy, a second court judgement finds in favour of a mobile phone user's head cancer claim against evidence from ICNIRP.

2020 5G begins to be rolled out around the world.

Switzerland halts the roll-out of **5G** pending further investigation of the health hazards.

In the USA, the Environmental Health Trust files against the **Federal Communications Commission** for its 'non-protective, inadequate and outdated wireless regulations.'

In the UK, leading human rights lawyer **Michael Mansfield QC** is reported to be heading the challenge to the British government over the health risks from **5G**.

In the USA and Canada, more communities reject the roll out of 5G on health grounds and more phones are pulled from the market on the grounds of failure to meet safety standards.

In Brussels, European Parliament members publish the first detailed report on conflicts of interest between **ICNIRP** and corporate interests in the mobile phone industry and the proposed roll out of **5G**.

1 One of Us is Mad

Brian Stein's Diary

I started using a mobile phone in about 1987. And for the next ten years or so there was no problem, there were no issues at all. In fact, I was one of those people who wanted more mobile phone masts, because the reception quality on the mobile wasn't good enough, particularly while in the car.

During 1999-2000 I started to notice some discomfort, a pain in my inner ear whilst I was on the mobile phone – specifically whilst I was on the phone. I took the phone away from my ear, the pain went away, brought the phone back, back came the pain. But with all the publicity surrounding mobile phones and the UK Health Protection Authority saying that it was perfectly safe, any problems were only temporary, I was assured and continued to use my mobile phone, although trying to cut down its use.

Then the discomfort I had been having after a period of time started to appear after shorter durations of time. I became concerned. I purchased an earpiece. I used the earpiece, but found no difference. I started to juggle around with the earpiece so that it was out of my ear, facing away from my ear, but it was all to no avail. When it was close to my ear, it caused me pain. And that pain gradually became more intense and came more quickly.

It was shortly after playing around with the earpiece that there was an article in WHICH Magazine. It said that using an earpiece might be worse than not using one, because it concentrated the microwaves, and certainly whether it was worse or slightly better I don't know, but it made no material difference.

Then during the summer of 2000 I started to notice a milder form of discomfort whilst I was on the hands free in the car.

I couldn't understand this, so again I tried to cut down on my mobile phone use whether it was to my head or hands free.

Then I started to notice some mild sensations when I simply had the mobile phone plugged in in the car. So I started to unplug my mobile in the car. I was concerned that there was something the matter with the unit, something the matter in the car. I was driving a Jaguar at the time, and I thought, I'm changing my car shortly, so if there's something wrong with the car it'll be improved with my new car.

I took delivery of my new car in September of 2000 – it was a 7 series BMW and I think looking back now it was the worst thing I could possibly have done. Top of the range 7 series, electronic everything, TV, CD, Satnav etc. It was full of gadgets. And my condition continued to get worse.

Then at the end of September 2000 I used my mobile phone for the last time. I put the phone to my head and the pain was excruciating. It was almost as if something in my inner ear had burst. The pain was so severe I couldn't bear the phone next to it. As soon as I put the phone to my ear the pain came back. As soon as I took the phone away the pain went away. But anywhere near my ear and the pain was becoming very, very severe.

At that stage I assumed that I was a freak. Other people seemed to have no problems at all, I was a one-off. I had never heard of electrical sensitivity and I assumed at that time that I had simply become sensitive to microchips in the mobile phone.

Within a number of weeks I realised it wasn't as simple as that. Because although I wasn't using a mobile phone, I noticed these weird sensations I'd started to get when I was in the car with the phone on hands free. I started to experience them around a computer, a television and indeed in my car when the satellite navigation system was turned on.

This gradually got worse, quite frightening, I became sensitive to the dishwasher and washing machine, and this was quite scary because I'd never heard of this happening before.

I was still concerned that the car I was driving wasn't right, the 7 series BMW. I suppose I hoped there was something wrong with the car, it was emitting a higher field than it should have done. I eventually made an appointment with a testing company, E.R.A Technologies in Leatherhead, Surrey, south of London to have the car checked out for electromagnetic fields. On 28 November, 2000, I drove down there, which was a bit worrying at the time, because the car was starting to affect me quite badly.

I got there and they conducted a number of tests and could find nothing the matter with the car. As I sat in the car I become quite sensitive to the car because I'd been in it a couple of hours driving, and when the satellite navigation system was turned on I could feel it quite badly. So it was then that I started to think, it's not the car. It's me, I'm the freak, I'm the one that's badly affected. I'm sensitive to microchips and I needed to remove them from my environment to help me to cope.

I started to live quite a restricted lifestyle. I stopped watching television, I stopped using a computer, I stopped being in the vicinity of computers, I stopped being in the house with the dishwasher on, with the washing machine on, and I started to remove microchips from my environment, both at home and at work.

I stopped using the BMW and I started using my wife's Nissan Micra, and the Micra was fine. I got another Micra as a precaution, and found that although the second Micra was the same style, the same age, it wasn't quite as good, so I continued using my wife's Micra thinking that I could get another car that would be better, in time. I subsequently found that each car I tried affected me after a period of time and I kept going back to relying on my wife's Nissan Micra.

I had to announce in work to a number of senior managers why I was driving a Nissan Micra and not my 7 Series BMW, because they were becoming concerned that I was about to seriously downgrade the company's car policy.

I then approached GTM Cars in Sutton Bonington about having a car built for me. They built a car with no microchips which

I thought would be fine for me. I obviously didn't understand enough because as soon as I got in the car and went out for a spin, the car was affecting me. It was a small car, a kit car, and much of the engine, the electrics, were relatively close to my body.

I realised that this wasn't as simple as microchips. It was more to do with other 'electromagnetic fields'. And indeed my wife went on the computer and found out about a condition called electrical sensitivity.

It was a condition that was recognised in Sweden, and it listed all sorts of conditions and I was able to tick the box for most of them. It became obvious quickly that I had become electrically sensitive and that I needed to take avoidance measures.

I went to my doctor and explained to him what had happened to me. This was in July 2001. I don't think he really believed me and he recommended a scan to reassure me although he didn't think I needed one because he didn't think there was anything the matter with me. But I was able to convince him that I wanted one and he was happy to put my name to a specialist.

I went to see a specialist but it was a waste of time. This was around September 2001. He didn't understand, he had no training in this area, his only view was, it can give headaches but there's nothing permanent. And if I thought it was the phone, and I'd stopped using it, that should be okay.

But the condition continued to worsen and I was beginning to become sensitive to other things. I could notice when someone had a mobile phone turned on nearby: although the effects became less dramatic, the number of different things that affected me increased and they became more dramatic.

I found a private hospital, the Breakspeare Hospital, that treated people who were chemically and electrically sensitive. I attended some tests and they gave me treatment – a course of tablets that I should take – rather expensive – but I took them. At one stage I suppose I was taking over one hundred tablets per day. I continued this for about nine months. Then I decided that was enough, it was making no difference to my condition, and I stopped taking the tablets and stopped attending the Breakspeare Hospital. I saw much evidence of people with chemical sensitivity and food allergies being helped at the hospital, but not ES.

Because of my condition I got in touch with one or two other people who were electrically sensitive. I became involved in ES-UK and the Radiation Research Trust, but I was still trying to keep a relatively low profile. My job as Chief Executive of Samworth Brothers involved my maintaining my credibility with the retailers, so being high profile in an area where the government was ridiculing and claiming it was psychosomatic was quite threatening to me as an individual and as a Chief Executive.

The volume of research I was seeing showing that low level non-ionising radiation was damaging to health helped me to understand that I wasn't a freak. I was the canary down the coal mine: an early warning signal of what was to come

I continued to keep a relatively low profile, and although gaining some influence in the electrically sensitive community, my name being passed on to journalists etc, I refused to be involved in any interviews. I'd seen one or two reports that had been made in local papers of people who were electrically sensitive and I wasn't very comfortable with it. They tended to be treated as freaks and they were just a sideshow as opposed to dealing with the issue, the science and the concerns that people should have been having for society, not just one or two people.

And then at the end of 2004 one or two things happened that made me start to speak out. Firstly a friend who knew of my condition suggested I should speak to a professor at Leicester University - so I thought, I'll give him a ring.

I plucked up courage and rang Professor Fothergill at Leicester University. I explained to him that I had become electrically sensitive and that a friend of a friend thought he might be interested: I lived nearby, I was a Chief Executive in Leicester, was he interested in doing any work with me, tests, analysis, experimentation?

After that I could hardly get a word in edgeways as Professor Fothergill told me he was ever so sorry, he was ever so busy, and he was ever so sorry, he was ever so busy, but he was really busy… and there was nothing he could do because he was ever so busy.

So before signing off I just asked him at the end of our conversation, what was his area of expertise. And he coughed and he spluttered and he told me that he was experimenting and doing research into 'the effects of electromagnetic fields on the human body'!

*When I put the phone down I literally knocked my head, thinking, here's a subject who is nearby, he's investigating this area and **he does not want to know me**.*

Bizarre.

You are a scientist. You research things. I am a citizen. We can help each other.

'One of us is mad,' I said to myself, 'I don't think it's me.'

2   A Brief History of The Diseases of Civilisation

Professor Fothergill's reluctance to engage with Brian Stein on the subject of electrosensitivity may have stemmed from the fact that there is a vast, disparate, but increasingly joined-up body of scientific, epidemiological and anecdotal evidence concerning the effects of electromagnetic fields and microwave radiation on living organisms.

This body of evidence dates back decades, even centuries, before mobile phones, ipads, tablets, masts and Wi-Fi, and what have become known as 'The Diseases of Civilisation'.

In 1868, G.M Beard, writing in the *Boston Medical and Surgical Journal*, noted 'neurasthenia, or nervous exhaustion' among telegraph workers in the USA. Nikola Tesla, the 'Father of electrical engineering', in later life displayed the signs of what would come to be termed 'electrohypersensitivity'. As his Pulitzer-prize-winning biographer described:

'The peculiar malady that now affected him was never diagnosed by the doctors who attended him. It was, however, an experience that nearly cost him his life. To doctors he appeared to at death's door... One of the symptoms of the illness was an acute sensitivity of all the sense-organs...this sensitivity was now so tremendously exaggerated that the effects were a form of torture. The ticking of a watch three rooms away sounded like the beat of hammers on an anvil. The vibration of ordinary city traffic, when transmitted through a chair or bench, pounded through his body.'

'It was necessary to place the legs of his bed on rubber pads to eliminate the vibrations. Ordinary speech sounded like thunderous pandemonium. The slightest touch had the mental effect of a tremendous blow... His pulse, he said, would vary from a few

feeble throbs per minute to more than one hundred and fifty. Throughout this mysterious illness he was fighting with a powerful desire to recover his normal condition...'

In 1928, workers at a General Electric plant in New York building an experimental radio transmitter complained of ill health. The main effect was heating, but when radiotherapy was, within two years, used in medical treatment, the side effects observed included were dizziness, nausea, weakness and sweating.

In 1932, the German doctor Erwin Schliephake coined the term 'electro-hypersensitivity' in data in the *German Medical Weekly* concerning patients experiencing unusual symptoms around radio towers at below thermal levels. He called this condition 'microwave' or 'radio wave sickness'. The symptoms Schliephake observed included severe headaches, fatigue, diminished sleep quality and lowered immune systems.

During the Second World War, with the operational deployment of radar (Radio Detecting and Ranging) using pulsed microwaves to detect enemy vessels and aircraft, the US Navy carried out studies showing symptoms of electrosensitivity and electrohypersensitivity in laboratory staff.

In 1960, Dr Allan Frey was a young neuroscientist working at General Electric's Advanced Electronics Center at Cornell University in the United States. A technician colleague said he could 'hear' radar. He asked Frey to check it out: 'And sure enough, I could hear it too,' Frey recalled. Frey started to document the Frey effect, which would suggest that non-thermal effects of radiofrequency radiation existed in addition to the accepted thermal effects of microwaves.

In the same year, the first semi-automatic private user car phone was launched in Sweden.

In 1967, the first popular microwave oven was marketed: its background was in radar technology. The vast majority of microwave oven users would be women, and most ovens would be located at breast height.

In 1972, in the USA, the race began between AT&T which owned Bell Labs and Motorola to build on the cumbersome and expensive car phones used by the police and a few thousand elite business types and develop the first portable mobile phone.

In the same year, a report (otherwise unpublicised) to the US Department of Defense stated that little was known about the possible health effects of repeated or long-term exposure to low levels of non-thermal radio frequency radiation of the types emitted by wireless communications devices.

In 1973, Martin Cooper of Motorola made the first cell (mobile) phone call – to a rival at Bell Labs, owned by AT&T. Motorola declared cell phones would be commercially available within three years, although no-one knew how to make this happen, and there was no network of microwave masts that would make it work.

In 1975, Allan Frey reported in *Annals of the New York Academy of Sciences* that non-thermal microwaves pulsed at certain modulations could induce dangerous 'leakage' in the barrier between the blood circulatory system and the brain of white rats. His method was to inject fluorescent dye into the circulatory system and sweep microwave frequencies across their bodies. Within minutes the dye had penetrated the rats' brains. He also stopped frogs' hearts dead with microwaves.

Frey was a member of the Institute of Electrical and Electronics Engineers (IEEE), which billed itself as 'a leading authority on areas ranging from aerospace systems, computers and telecommunications to biomedical engineering, electric power and consumer electronics.' Both Frey and Dr Louis Slesin noted that the IEEE committees that set microwave radiation safety levels were dominated by companies such as Raytheon, General Electric, the telecommunications industry and now the cell phone industry. Private sector interests were dictating public health policy, and with increasingly vast profits to be made, the so-called 'safe' radiation thresholds were far higher than Frey and Slesin thought they should be.

Frey's non-thermal microwave findings caused uproar in neuroscience and led to his being threatened by the US government with the withdrawal of his funding from the Office of Naval Research. Scientists were hired and funded by the Pentagon to 'war-game' or replicate his research and claimed to have failed to do so: but did not disclose their methodology. Frey was advised to pursue other lines of inquiry if he wanted to go on receiving funding, and suspended his research.

Om P. Gandhi and his team at the University of Utah, meanwhile, conducted Defense Department and telecommunications industry-funded research showing the effects of microwaves on the cognitive functions of rats on which the American National Standards Institute (ANSI) set industry safety standards.

In 1976, in the USA, the first of three studies by epidemiologist Dr Samuel Milham of Washington State Department of Health was published by the National Institute of Occupational Safety and Health (NIOSH). The study showed that, between 1950 and 1971, Washington state firefighters had increased mortality due to brain cancer, malignant melanoma, and non-Hodgkin's lymphoma. As Milham observed: *'None of these cancers had an intuitive connection to inhaled carcinogens.'*

In 1979, the *Saturday Review* in the United States carried the story *'The Invisible Threat: The Stifled Story of Electric Waves'*, describing the adverse health effects of electromagnetic fields and microwave radiation on people living on and near military bases. The article described how scientists on whose research the revelations were based were vilified and their laboratories closed down.

In particular it detailed how, between 1953 and 1976, the US Embassy in Moscow had been irradiated by the Soviets with microwaves only one five hundredth the power of safety levels that would be set by the mobile phone industry in the 1990s, yet with serious long term health consequences for embassy staff. The State Department had decided not to inform embassy staff that the building was being irradiated, and in 1970 carried out a secret study codenamed 'Project Pandora'. The study allegedly concluded that there were no negative health effects from the irradiation; the data however on which it was based was destroyed. Ambassador Walter J Stoessel, meanwhile, who had served two years in the Moscow Embassy and suffered ill-health during this period, died of leukaemia ten years later at the age of sixty-six.

In 1980, in the USA, Dr Louis Slesin founded *Microwave News,* which would become the independent benchmark for monitoring the mobile phone industry.

In 1983, the first commercially available 'brick' cell phones with a battery life of half an hour were rolled out in the USA at US $4,000 apiece. They would soon become the yuppie weapon of choice. Since they were 'non-thermal' – they did not produce heat – cell phones were presumed to be free from biological effects on humans and their invisible radio frequency signals were apparently not subjected to safety testing, either by the industry or by agencies of government.

In fact, Mays Swicord of the University of Maryland and the Food & Drug Administration had produced research showing that the same radio frequency proposed for cell phones could disturb the DNA within human brain cells. Swicord would remain at the FDA for another decade.

In 1985, in the USA, based on the work of Om P. Gandhi and others, ANSI had continuously lowered recommended safety levels. This led ANSI to fear litigation in future and withdraw from the field. Its place was taken up by the Institute for Electronics and Electrical Engineering (IEEE).

In 1986, Carl Blackman was a bioelectromagnetic expert who had worked at the US Environmental Protection Agency since 1970. Blackman's findings regarding the biological effects of non-thermal electromagnetic fields confirmed and extended the work of Allan Frey and others, troubling him and the EPA to the point where the latter halted his research altogether.

The Fate of the Ericsson Technicians

In 1988, in Sweden, outside Stockholm, Per Segerback, a technician with Ericsson's Ellemtel research and development team, experienced the first symptoms of electrical hypersensitivity. Segerback had been part of the young, enthusiastic generation of 'techies' trained at university in Uppsala and then in California's Silicon Valley, where he learned about micropressors and semiconductors. He was also one of the first in Sweden to work with high resolution colour VDTs from England.

The symptoms were like something out of a sci-fi horror movie: stinging and burning sensations in his face, sleeplessness, anxiety and red patches over his body. Tested hormonally for conventional stress levels, he measured averagely: this was something different. Worse, in addition to the VDTs, he began reacting in the same way to fluorescent lights, electrical equipment in his home, even to electromagnetic fields in his car. He took to long walks at night and sleeping in his car with the ignition off.

'It sure was cold,' he recalled, but preferred not to speak further of this period, 'I have repressed it.'

More than fifty young Ericsson technicians experienced similar symptoms to greater and lesser degrees. The company's initial reaction towards its employees was concerned and protective: some took sick leave and Ericsson sought and received government funds to investigate the phenomenon. The company parked an aluminium camper van outside Segerback's house so that he had an electrically-free place to sleep. They 'sanitised' a room in the Segerback house from electromagnetic fields with iron sheeting. At work, they built him a similar iron-clad room and Segerback commuted between these two rooms in an elderly taxi in which he could sit as far away as possible from the vehicle's electronics, during which journeys the driver would disable the electronic fare meter.

Ericsson's initial reaction would change, however: the technicians were, in the words of Swedish journalist Gunni Nordstrom, 'more or less silenced', with the exception, it seemed, of Segerback. Four years later, in 1993, while still employed in his heavily 'sanitised' office, he gave Nordstrom an interview.

'My skin still hurts when I am exposed to electricity,' he told her, 'I get blotchy red. It is terrible and hurts a lot more than it might appear to. When my computer broke recently I had to use another which was temporarily placed closer than the ordinary one and I felt it right away. It means there is a lot of direct radiation from the computer itself.'

'My eldest son, who is twelve, is often sad, but Anna, two, has never experienced anything except my illness so she takes it naturally. When we are together she runs ahead and turns off electricity everywhere.'

Electrical hypersensitivity was not yet recognised by traditional medicine in Sweden and two skin doctors and a stress researcher had recommended that Ellemtel should not carry out electrical sanitisation, as they did not believe electricity had anything to do with the problem. Segerback, however, was convinced.

'We technicians at Ellemtel know that electric sanitation is the only thing that helps,' he told Nordstrom.

Segerback was clearly a sufficiently valuable asset for Ericsson and Ellemtel to want to retain his services, and Segerback himself needed to work to support his family. What he couldn't or wouldn't tell Nordstrom was what had happened to the other 'more or less silenced' Ericsson technicians.

The interview was conducted in the presence of an Ericsson/ Ellemtel minder. There was more at stake here for Ericsson – a rising player in global telecommunications - than the welfare of one of its most valuable - and best-informed - employees.

*

Meanwhile, in 1992, the IEEE in the USA had lowered safety standards for general public exposure to cell phone emissions to a level five times less than a decade earlier. Their yardstick was still the work of Om P. Gandhi.

In January, 1993, David Reynard, in Florida, brought the first American cancer and mobile phone-related lawsuit against the NEC cell phone company, following the death of his wife from what he asserted was a wireless radiation-aggravated brain tumour. Mobile phone stocks plummetted. Tom Wheeler, president of the Cellular Communications and Internet Association (CTIA) in America, announced that the CTIA was going to fund a comprehensive $28.5 million research programme that would prove that mobile phones were safe.

Wheeler commissioned and funded epidemiologist and law graduate George Carlo to carry out the programme. Wheeler saw Carlo as a safe bet. Carlo had already supplied industry-funded studies asserting that breast implants were only a minimal health risk and that low levels of dioxin (as used in Agent Orange) were not dangerous. By 1995, Carlo had reputedly set to work on the Wireless Technology Research project (WTR).

INIRC (International Non-ionising Radiation Committee) became ICNIRP (International Committee on Non-Ionising Radiation Protection). The new body was again populated by representatives of the mobile phone industry.

By 1993, there were 15 million cell phones in the USA. The Food & Drug Administration acknowledged in an internal memo that studies suggested a link between non-thermal microwave radiation and increased cancer risk. Again, the memo was largely unnoticed/ignored.

By 1994, there were 90 million mobile phones worldwide.

Dr Henry Lai, a biophysicist at the University of Washington, and Narendra P. Singh were beginning to make discoveries about the effects of microwave frequencies on the structure of rat DNA. Modulated electromagnetic radiation could cause breaks in the DNA strands that might lead to genetic damage and mutations with potential consequences for generations – all this being the consequence of a single two-hour exposure.

The Food & Drug Administration, meanwhile, approved cell phones for general use without safety testing. Shortly afterwards, Mays Swicord left the FDA to join Motorola.

Motorola, alarmed by the Reynard lawsuit, reassured stockholders and went on the attack, targeting and attempting to discredit Henry Lai. Industry-commissioned 'war-gaming' studies by Motorola-funded scientists claimed to 'fail to replicate' Lai's genotoxic findings: the suggestion being that his was 'bad' science. This was the tactic that would set the ringtone for the cell phone operators' battle for hearts and minds around the world over the next two and half decades.

Henry Lai meanwhile went on to review 350 studies and find that around 50% reported biological effects from electromagnetic radiation emitted by cell phones. But only 25% of industry-funded studies reported as such – as opposed to 75% of independently-funded studies.

In 1996, in the USA, the new Telecommunications Act was passed, after nearly US $50 million worth of lobbying and 'donations' from the cell phone industry. Section 704 of the Act – signed by President Clinton – specifically prohibited citizens and local governments from stopping the construction of cell towers on the grounds of health concerns.

By the end of the year, telecom companies had paid the federal government more than US $8 billion for portions of microwave frequency. Cell phone antennae sprang up across the country on apartment buildings, church steeples, streetlights, fire and clock towers and flagpoles, in parks and along highways. Frequently unnoticed, the wireless age had entered community public space - and the home.

Professor Om P. Gandhi produced a paper which concluded that microwave exposure into the brains of children turned the accepted safety standards for cell phones on their heads. The industry's reaction was swift – it cut off Gandhi's funding and set out to discredit him.

In 1997, in the USA, when Motorola-funded scientist Jerry Phillips successfully replicated Henry Lai's findings showing negative health effects from non-thermal radiation, the company including Mays Swicord put him under pressure to alter his conclusion. Phillips lost his job at Motorola and his Defense Department-related research funding.

The Food & Drug Administration, having acknowledged that several studies suggested a link between microwave radiation and increased cancer risk, now stated: *'Little is known about the possible health effects of repeated or long-term exposure to low levels of radio frequency radiation (RFR) of the types emitted by wireless communications devices.'*

In Sweden, the government-sponsored Council for Work Life Research (RALF) inquiry began into electrosensitivity.

At the Karolinska Institute in Stockholm, where the Nobel Prize for Medicine was awarded, neuroscientist Professor Olle Johansson and former environmental manager for Swedish telecom company Ericsson, Orjan Hallberg, were investigating possible links between the recent proliferation of microwave PCs and a decline in health in the Swedish population. Johansson had been studying electromagnetic hypersensitivity since 1985. Their findings gave rise for concern.

In 1998, the ICNIRP EU industry safety standards were laid down. In the same year, Tice and Hook's findings were published concerning DNA breakage caused by prolonged exposure to microwave radiation.

By 1999, there were 200 million mobile phone users worldwide. In February of that year, George Carlo presented the findings of his $28.5 million industry-funded WTR programme to Tom Wheeler and the heads of the Cellullar Technology and Internet Association and CEOs of American mobile industry providers including AT&T, Apple and Motorola.

In a closed-door session, Carlo told them that the fifty studies commissioned by WTR and reviews of many more raised 'serious questions' about mobile phone safety. After ten minutes, according to Carlo, Wheeler cut him off: 'That's enough, George,' he said. Carlo was bundled from the building to a waiting car by two burly security men, one of whom confided he had until recently been in the employ of the US Secret Service.

Carlo did not give up. In October of that year, he wrote to cell phone industry CEOs repeating the fact that WTR's research had found the risk of 'rare neuroepithelial tumours on the outside of the brain was more than doubled' and that there appeared to be a correlation between 'brain tumours occurring on the right side of the head and the use of the phone on the right side of the head'. He added that 'the ability of radiation from a phone's antenna to cause functional genetic damage (was) definitely positive.'

He urged wireless industry CEOs to give the public 'the information they need to make an informed judgement', adding that some of their number had 'repeatedly and falsely claimed that wireless phones are safe for all consumers including children.'

In other words, for *cell phones*, read *cancer cell phones*.

Tom Wheeler of the CTIA had already had Carlo muscled out of the building. Now he wasted no time in shooting the messenger. He rubbished Carlo in the media and suggested that the WTR studies had not been published in peer-reviewed journals (in spite of the fact that according to Carlo, Carlo had repeatedly briefed Wheeler and his colleagues on the findings and the latter would be published in peer review journals).

Dr Louis Slesin of *Microwave News* in New York was an experienced Carlo-watcher. Slesin had no brief for Tom Wheeler and the CTIA, but he was sceptical about Carlo, whom he regarded as self-serving, and even as to whether or not the WTR studies actually existed. Slesin would go on to describe Carlo as less a messenger who had been shot, than a 'jilted lover' whom Wheeler didn't need any more.

Either way, Wheeler's tactics of keeping the argument going instead of extinguishing it, and committing the industry's burgeoning resources to commissioning further industry-friendly studies while rubbishing the finding of independent scientists, would continue: and there would be plenty of scientists ready and willing to take the wireless industry's coin.

In the USA, Om P. Gandhi stepped down from heading the safety standards committee of IEEE and was succeeded by C.K Chou of the City of Hope Hospital.

In 2000, in February, in Switzerland, the Federal Council issued Ordinance relating to Protection from Non-ionising Radiation, applying the 'precautionary principle' regarding wireless radiation that would be advocated in the UK by Sir William Stewart.

In March, in Sweden, RALF publicly convened to hear the EHS evidence. But the outcome was a disappointment to the providers of 33 statements and 414 letters whose testimony was given just over one page in RALF's report to the Swedish government: a report that concluded in principal that Electrical Hypersensitivity did not exist. The contributors decided to compile their own evidence for independent publication.

In April, 2000, the Ecolog Institute study was sponsored by mobile phone operator T–Mobil in Germany. The report, which analysed dozens of peer-reviewed studies, concluded: *'Given the results of the present epidemiological studies, it can be concluded that electromagnetic fields with frequencies in the mobile telecommunications range do play a role in the development of cancer.'*

'This is particularly notable for tumours of the central nervous system.'

The Ecolog report also recommended that existing safety thresholds on radiation exposure should be cut to 1/1000th of those currently in force.

T-Mobil, confronted with this conclusion, buried the Ecolog study and commissioned a further study suggesting there was no problem. Years later, the original Ecolog study was leaked by a T-Mobil employee (**for a link to the original Ecolog study see Appendix 5.**)

There were now 100 million cell phone users in the USA.

The US Food & Drug Administration officially advised the National Toxicology Program: *'There is currently insufficient scientific basis for concluding either that wireless communication technologies are safe or that they pose a risk to millions of users. A significant research effort, involving large, well-planned animal experiments, is needed to provide the basis to assess the risk to human health of wireless communications devices.'*

Thorsten Ritz's study showed that the magnetic compass in birds was disrupted even by electromagnetic frequencies well below ICNIRP safety thresholds.

Franz Adlkofer's team started the REFLEX project. The study concluded that DNA could be damaged by electromagnetic radiation and triggered an alert tone within the mobile phone industry.

In November, 2000, Dr Gerard Hyland of the Department of Physics at the University of Warwick published his findings regarding the biological effects of mobile phone masts in the *Lancet*. Dr Hyland had already reported his findings to the Science and Technology Committee at the House of Commons in Westminster and would go on to report them to the European Parliament.

Dr Hyland's principal concern was with research which had found that existing safety thresholds failed to address the possibility of adverse health effects on living organisms. He cited the case of an epileptic child living near a mast base station, whose seizures increased from two a month to an average of eight a day when close to the mast. He reported a similar pattern with other children suffering from headaches and nosebleeds.

Dr Hyland also reported findings of reduced growth in pine trees, chromosomal and reproductive damage in plants and a six-fold increase in chromosome damage in cows. He concluded that the occurrence of adverse health effects in the case of animals indicated that the effects of operating masts were real and not psychosomatic.

Could pine trees pretend? Did plants dissimulate? Might cows be imagining things?

It seemed not. Yet, ten years on, the 'psychological' explanation would still be purveyed by Dr Michael Repacholi of ICNIRP, the UK Health Protection Agency and Dr James Rubin of King's College London.

At the end of 2000, Brian Stein became electrically sensitive, having been reassured by the UK Health Protection Agency that there was no evidence of harm to the general population.

*

Sir William Stewart's Report was published on Wireless Communication. Among many recommendations, Stewart, the Government Scientific Advisor, proposed that the use of mobile phones by children be restricted:

'If there are currently unrecognised adverse health effects from the use of mobile phones, children may be more vulnerable because of their developing nervous system, the greater absorption of energy in the tissues of the head, and a longer lifetime of exposure.'

Stewart's findings became known as 'the Precautionary Principle'. In the same year, the British government auctioned £22.5 billion worth of 3G wireless bandwidth to mobile phone operators.

By 2001, there were 500 million mobile phone users worldwide.

The European Standard method was introduced for measuring the Specific Absorption Rate (SAR) - or how much radio wave energy a body received from a particular mobile phone. These rates varied from phone to phone, but *'All models sold in the UK already meet international exposure guidelines.'*

C.K Chou, in the United States, while remaining in post at IEEE, took up a senior position with Motorola. In spite of what would appear to be a conflict of interests, Chou's appointment was accepted by IEEE. Chou proceeded to apply pressure to relax the exposure standards for cell phones, contrary to the findings of Om P. Gandhi.

In 2002, in the USA, Gandhi was told that he would lose his industry funding if he went on reporting that children were more at risk from exposure than adults, and insisting that the industry's safety thresholds should be tightened again.

Chou also tried to place an article criticising Gandhi's research models. Four scientists described Chou's critique of Gandhi as 'scientific junk' and the editor of the magazine refused to publish it.

The UK Department of Health issued *'Mobile 'Phones and Health'* in the wake of the Stewart Report: *'On the advice of the Stewart Group further major research, funded by the government and the mobile phone industry, is now being undertaken.'*

The language was cautious: *'Radio waves emitted above a certain level can cause heating effects in the body. International guidelines seek to ensure that exposure is kept below that level. All mobile phones sold in the UK meet these guidelines.'*

'The balance of current research evidence suggests that exposure to radio waves below levels set out in international guidelines do not cause health problems for the general population. However, there is some evidence that changes in brain activity can occur below these guidelines, but it isn't clear why. There are significant gaps in our scientific knowledge…'

The Department of Health appeared to endorse Sir William Stewart's 'Precautionary Principle': keep calls short, discourage young children from using mobile phones. The Department also issued the leaflet *'Mobile Phone Base Stations and Health'*.

'Eight old-school secretaries don't fall apart at the same time!'

In Sweden, dissatisfied with the lack of government reaction to their testimonies, the RALF action group members independently published their personal accounts of electrical hypersensitivity. The accounts, many by highly-educated professionals, went back as far as the 1980s.

As despatches from the everyday life of a technology-based society, they made disturbing reading: skin problems, headaches and visual and mental impairment, throbbing in teeth with amalgam fillings, bitter saliva and lassitude, nausea, joint pains, sleeplessness and shortness of breath, often in clusters of people – *'Eight old-school secretaries don't fall apart at the same time!'* - with common recurring features including prolonged exposure to computer screens, especially when employers installed more powerful upgrades with front-mounted magnetic coils, use of cordless phones, cell phones and proximity to base stations and fluorescent lamps.

The consequences among the contributors included increased sensitivity even to less powerful electrical sources such as TV sets, microwave ovens and electric lamps, domestic heating pipes and electric cables, compounded by municipal rejection, employer disbelief/outright hostility, redundancy, the struggle for disability benefits, economic hardship, relationship deterioration and breakdown, ongoing anxiety, social isolation and misery.

A recurring theme was the ineffectiveness of the 'psychological' explanation and cognitive behavioural therapy as a remedy. As one contributor testified:

'Do you think that within a period of a few years I would agree to moving four times, losing all our life's savings – the savings that others of our age see as security for when they get older – if I wasn't convinced of what it is my wife suffers from? I don't need any scientific proof. She is proof enough.'

'Due to all the other moves and extra costs since 1993, when my wife was afflicted with electro-hypersensitivity, we have lost about one and a half million Swedish Crowns. You probably understand that that is not something one just gives away. We once had the dream of moving to France when we got older. That money would have been the key to realising that dream.'

Others: *'I am 33 years old now, longing to be a mother, longing to settle down with my boyfriend. Those are my dreams. My reality is quite another.'*

'My body and my psyche are completely worn out... My reality is unreal. My boyfriend and I are looking for a house, and that requires an environment that is almost impossible to find.'

And: *'Today, I can't be at home at certain times because of this without getting very sick. So where am I supposed to go? Run around from place to place to keep from getting to sick? There will soon be nowhere my body can recuperate, and in that case, how long will my body be able to keep on going? The situation is very oppressive.'*

Was this real or the collective neurosis of a developed society?

'For the past few days I have been sleeping in the car beneath a large rock on a beach in Spain...'

'In the wintry-cold Sweden of 1997, I had to flee out into the forest and sleep in an unheated trailer, while at the same time I was afflicted with symptoms of paralysis in my arms and legs, problems with breathing, vomiting, unable to go to the toilet without help etc. Since I was afraid that the hardships would kill me and was close to having my fingers and toes frostbitten, my boyfriend and I were forced to take the risk that I might not be able to take an airline flight and fled out of the country.'

'We found an isolated place in radio shadow on one of the Canary Islands...'

Back in Sweden, some relief was afforded through the removal of amalgam dental fillings, expensive vitamins, protective clothing and EMF reduction in the home, often with the help of a sympathetic electrician/technician – and in some cases retreat to a car, trailer, boat, cabin or even tent in the woods. But this was accompanied by ongoing social exclusion and constant fear – frequently realised - that the growing number of wireless masts would force further dislocation.

This was the life of the electro-refugee: *'I'm on the street again and can't hold out much longer...'*

'I have changed addresses eight times, five of which during the last year. It is truly a question of being a refugee in your own country...'

'I do not have the slightest doubt that the problem is real...'

'The worst of it all is not being believed by doctors...'

'I left there in tears, feeling very degraded...'

'What kind of life is this? Is it a life?'

'I try to keep on going for the sake of my children, otherwise suicide would have been an easier way out of this hell...'

'Suicide...'

'Suicide...'

This was a real-life horror movie, complete with the plotline where those in possession of the truth were isolated by an Orwellian disbelief in their situation and overridden by commercial interests, while those in authority refused to confront the issue. This was a 21st century equivalent of tobacco and asbestos – except that electromagnetic fields were imposed on, and not voluntarily inhaled by, the user - and nobody as yet was talking about cancer.

The book containing these testimonies was published in Sweden – three years would pass before an English translation became available on a limited scale. By this time, Swedish government and industry attitudes would have shifted from the 'EHS does not exist' position while British attitudes had hardened in favour of the status quo.

Why Sweden? Why were people not having their amalgam fillings replaced and moving to cars, trailers, boats, cabins and tents all over Europe? Or were they?

*

In Finland, Professor Dariusz Leszczynski's study for the Finnish government confirmed the findings of Allan Frey and Leif Salford regarding the biological impact of low levels of pulsed mobile phone signals on the blood-brain barrier. The study made headlines around the world. The CTIA responded that 'more research is needed.'

Dr Gro Harlem Brundtland, former Prime Minister of Norway and Director-General of the World Health Organisation, told a Norwegian reporter she had banned mobile phones from her office in Geneva because she became ill if one was brought within about four metres (13 feet) of her.

This news, published on March 9, 2002 in *Dagbladet*, was ignored by every other newspaper in the world, but not by her WHO subordinate Dr Michael Repacholi, who was in charge of the International EMF Project and was closely associated with the mobile phone industry. Repacholi responded with a public statement belittling her concerns.

Dr Brundtland, a physician trained in public health, was subsequently heavily criticised for 'scaring people from using cell phones' as she put it, and 'telling the truth about my illness' the origins of which she attributed to an accident with a microwave oven in her home. Five months later, for reasons that many suspected were related to her statement about cell phones, Dr Brundtland announced she would step down from her leadership post at the WHO after just one term - allegedly unseated by Repacholi.

Alasdair Philips was scientific director of Powerwatch, an organisation that researched electromagnetic fields. He was also a director of EMFields, which sold 'electrosmog' detectors or acoustimeters with which Philips and others could 'sweep' homes and workplaces for levels of microwave radiation and advise on how these could be reduced – as he would do in the case of Brian Stein.

Philips contributed to an article in *The Engineer* magazine on electrosensitivity and the technology available to help electrically sensitive people. The article cited the case of advertising photographer Faisal Khawaja, an otherwise healthy and active young man who had become electrically sensitive after suffering acute headaches, dizziness and cognitive impairment whenever he used his mobile phone.

Referred by his GP for tests for a brain tumour, Khawaja was pronounced healthy and advised to take paracetamol. When this had no effect, and with his career in jeopardy – 'as in any other modern industry, advertising is dependent on technology' - Khawaja left London for Buckinghamshire, only to find a microwave mast being erected outside his house.

*

In 2003, Swedish neurosurgeon Leif Salford at the Rausing Laboratory picked up on Allan Frey's work and confirmed his findings. Salford found that microwave exposure killed rodents' brain cells and stimulated neurons associated with Alzheimer's disease: 'A rat's brain is very much the same as a human's,' he told the BBC, 'They have the same blood-brain barrier and neurons. We have good reason to believe that what happens in rats' brains also happens in humans… a whole generation of (mobile phone) users may suffer negative effects in middle age.'

In Athens, 2G and 3G mobile phones likewise disrupted the cognitive functions of Lukas H. Margaritis's rats.

In the UK, the EM Radiation Research Trust was founded at Westminster by solicitor Mike Bell and cancer survivor Eileen O'Connor, as a result of the Stewart Report, with the aim of building relationships with industry, governments and regulators in the UK and Europe. Sir William Stewart was appointed Chairman of the UK Health Protection Agency.

In 2004, in Poland, the Bortkiewicz study revealed sleep disturbance and loss of concentration in people living close to microwave masts.

In the USA, Dr Samuel Milham's study of male breast cancer in office workers exposed to high levels of electromagnetic fields and radio frequency radiation was published by NIOSH: *'This added to an already impressive body of reports linking male breast cancer to EMF and RFR. This cancer is so rare that its repeated appearance in EMF/RFR exposure situations functions like a sentinel cancer for these exposures.'*

Anne Silk had retired from a successful career as an optician in London's Wimpole Street. She had set up a practice at home, where she worked amid a battery of Japanese and American equipment generating powerful magnetic fields: 'And I got very electrosensitive... *susceptible*, as we should say. I started getting the sensation of putting a sharp nail into your ear and out again. It was excruciating for a microsecond. I started getting migraines.'

Silk combined her personal experience of electrosensitivity with her scientific background to research a series of academic papers addressing the subject in a wider context. In October 2004, she spoke on 'Migraine Equivalent – An Explanation for Electrosensitivity' in Prague, Czech Republic:

'In interviewing over 80 people who considered themselves to be electrically sensitive, it should be noted that the majority attributed the start of their problems to fluorescent light installation, at home or at work, and tubes of which are well known to flicker at mains frequency and harmonics. Also, although many reported childhood migraine, they all said they had grown out of it...'

*'ES people are often diagnosed with Fybromyalgia and with this condition patients show increased sensitivity to mechanical, thermal **and electrical** stimuli; once central sensitization has occurred, only minimal nociceptive input is required to maintain the sensitised state and clinical pain.'*

'Could it be that ES, which has been masquerading as a 'challenge to conventional wisdom'... is all the time lurking in the background as a ME/V?... All migrainous conditions are paroxysmal disorders caused by electrical overload in the brain, and sensory overload in a previously stressed system can, in a percentage of people, trigger a wide range of symptoms with remarkable parallels to those reported in ES.'

Silk was a respected medical scientific professional who would sit on Department of Health and Health Protection Agency committees and become the first woman 'Master' of her City of London Livery Company. She had a string of letters after her name longer than many UK government scientists and medical officers. If there was such a thing as 'the establishment', Silk was a pillar. Yet she despaired of the attitude of British scientists and General Practitioners towards electrosensitivity and possible biological health hazards from electromagnetic fields:

'My figure of speech for scientists is, we've got a school and we've got steep steps coming down from it, and some children are falling down breaking their legs. And they carry on. And nobody looks at the steps.'

'Why do the medical profession refuse to believe certain things? I learned this years ago. It is because the mantra is, 'If we haven't taught you it, it doesn't exist.' 'We've taught you everything – if we haven't taught you it, it isn't there. So don't listen to a word.'

May the Force Be With You

In the UK, Chief Inspector Stephen Strong and five other people at North Walsham police station in Norfolk had been experiencing dizziness and severe headaches. A Tetra microwave mast had recently been installed at the station. Chief Inspector Strong was told by police medical officers that he was imagining things.

Brian Stein read the item in the press:

Around about this time I read in the newspaper about a Chief Inspector Strong who had become ill, along with one or two other people in the police station after they had installed a Tetra mast. So I eventually got the telephone number of the station. I tried a few times and didn't get him, but after a while I got through to Chief Inspector Strong.

Because he'd been in the press, I asked the question, is that Chief Inspector Strong who's been in the paper as a result of suffering from the Tetra mast? And I immediately had a very aggressive, very defensive Chief Inspector Strong on the 'phone, saying, 'What do you want to know for?' Are you the press?'

And my response was: 'No no, calm down, my name's Brian Stein, I'm the Chief Executive of Samworth Brothers and the only reason I'm ringing you is I'm electrically sensitive. I understand what you're going through and I'm ringing simply to give you some advice: because if you continue to work in that environment you will become severely electrically sensitive like me and then there will be no going back. You need to be very careful.'

And within that 60 seconds of saying that to him, this rough, gruff Chief Inspector Strong went from being rough and gruff to being virtually on the edge of tears as he explained to me how he had been a star in the force and as a result of becoming electrically sensitive he had become 'a bum' and he was going to probably retire from the force.

They had given him an ultimatum – they wouldn't move him to another station, they'd investigated him, they'd had him checked out by a doctor, there was nothing the matter with him, he was imagining it, so he either got back to work or he retired. So the force was trying to do a deal with him where he would retire on full pension on the understanding that he didn't go to the press.

He explained that as soon as he got away from the police station and went home his condition slowly went away and he was fine and as soon as he came back to the station all these weird sensations started again, but there were also a number of other people at the station who were the same.

He knew what was causing it, he knew the effects, he knew how dramatic it was and he knew he had to get away from it, which was why he was negotiating his retirement, so there was no real advice I could give him, I think he'd worked it out for himself.

He was on the point of despair at having to give up his job that he'd loved. Because they wouldn't move the mast. And privately he said that, in a one to one conversation with one of the engineers, they'd admitted that they'd installed the mast too low. But the engineer wasn't going to repeat that with witnesses.

Incidentally, when I 'phoned the Chief Inspector a few years later, he hadn't retired. They had removed the mast and he was able to continue working.

But this was something that made me think long and hard. The police force had tried to cover it up, to buy him off on condition he didn't go to the press. They obviously had a problem, but it was too delicate to deal with. Again this was of concern to me, along with the conclusion that Professor Fothergill wasn't interested in researching the subject seriously.

*

Stein no longer used a mobile phone, had traded in his £50,000 BMW 7 Series for his wife's Nissan Micra with 200,000 miles on the clock, avoided computers, did not watch TV, go to the cinema or listen to music from devices connected to the mains, and switched off the mains electricity at home at night.

Most electrically sensitive people he knew had had to give up their jobs. At his job, where he had grown the Samworth Brothers food business from £100 million to £500 million, he could control his environment and use flip charts and a hands-free speakerphone. At home, by contrast, he could not enjoy many of the fruits and conveniences of success. As a lifelong supporter of Liverpool FC, many of whose matches he had attended in England and abroad, the lack of access to their television appearances was particularly painful.

Brian Stein's Diary

I'd been to the Land Rover agents in Melton, trying to get an old Land Rover. I'd spoken to the sales director and asked him to get me an old car. I explained to him I was electrically sensitive and he wanted to know why and what the sensations were like. I said, you don't want to know. He said no, I'm interested. I asked him why and he said he was starting to get some weird sensations himself whilst he was on the mobile phone, and headaches. And it was concerning him. So I said, cut down on your mobile phone. He said it was impossible, his job was just so much on the mobile phone.

I warned him if you don't, you'll end up like me and you'll regret it for the rest of your life, it's a very restrictive lifestyle.

He took it on board, except I don't think he did and when I had a phone call from them to come and look at a car they'd got for me (which was totally inappropriate) one of the sales people showed it to me and he was in the background. There he was, on his mobile phone. And I had to smile to myself, it was obvious my warnings had had little impact with him. And I thanked them for their efforts and departed.

But subsequently I had some conversations with some Swedish people who were recommending an old Volvo or a Land Rover, but needed to be diesel, their argument being that if you get an old one and it's a diesel there are fewer EMFs. This was nine months later. So I went back to the Land Rover agency in Melton and the person I had seen previously was gone. A lady had replaced him and I had a chat with her. I explained my condition again and what I was looking for and she explained that with the Land Rover, even with the early diesel, they were full of microchips. This rather depressed me.

In the course of having a chat with her about the issue, I explained that I had been in previously and spoken to her predecessor. She said it was a bit sad about him. I asked why and she said he'd died a number of months earlier. Oh, what did he die of? He died of a brain tumour.

This was a guy in his early forties.

She said that the hospital were concerned about his mobile phone use. As were the family.

So I added those three things together, the police, the professor, somebody dying in their early forties of a brain tumour having told me they were getting headaches using their mobile phone, and although adding them together didn't prove anything, with my own condition it was an indicator that something wasn't right. It caused brain tumours, it caused electrical sensitivity. The authorities were not interested and the professors were intimidated from doing work in this area. And that's when I decided that I really must speak out. I wouldn't be able to live with myself if in five, ten, twenty years' time, however long it took, they eventually realised that mobile phones, microwaves, caused brain tumours and I'd done nothing to speak out.

In January 2005, in the UK, Brian Stein, having told his colleagues in the Samworth Brothers boardroom about his electrosensitivity, 'came out' in an interview with Nic Fleming of the *Daily Telegraph*.

The experience as Stein recalled was 'liberating and distressing… exposing yourself as a nutcase.'

'*Medical people treat me as if I've just told them I'm visiting Earth from the moon,*' he told Fleming, '*I suspect that in 20 years we will have a problem that will make the issue of asbestos pale into insignificance.*'

'Scientists and health advisers are taking the claims of people who say electricity makes them ill seriously for the first time,' said the *Telegraph*. The piece cited the work of Sir William Stewart, the upcoming Essex Trials, the UK Health Protection Agency and Professor Olle Johansson at the Karolinska Institute in Stockholm, who said: *'If you put a radio near a source of EMFs you will get interference. The human brain has an electric field, so if you put sources of EMFs nearby, it is not surprising that you get interference, interaction with systems and damage to cells and molecules.'*

Brian Stein's Diary, 2005

The article went out on 24 January 2005. And after that I had every single newspaper and television channel ringing me wanting to do interviews. I decided I would do the TV channels, I'd do the local papers, the radio channels. I'd make myself available for one week and that was it.

And interestingly enough, after the first article Gill Meara from the UK Health Protection Agency commented on the radio that it was all a load of rubbish. After a fair bit of debate, and debate and debate, amongst the media, the next interview was a little more conciliatory, and then towards the end of the week the attitude of Gill Meara on the local radio was along the lines of, we need to help these people who are electrically sensitive. The UK Health Protection Agency had learned that there was sympathy from the general public and the media towards ES people.

So I thought that was a victory, I thought that was quite a concession from the Health Protection Agency, saying that they needed to help these people. I felt that I'd done my bit at that moment in time and I could watch now and see what they did.

The truth was they used and abused whatever information they had to deny, to ridicule, to pinpoint any research they possibly could that showed that it didn't exist, whilst ridiculing any research that showed that it did. And that was true not just of electrical sensitivities but studies into brain tumours, cancer, cell damage and other things. The UK Health Protection Agency, that I thought was there to protect my health, I very quickly realised was there to protect the mobile phone industry and the economy, and to devise a strategy to ensure that the sympathy towards ES people was destroyed.

Some consequences of the article were more unexpected than others: *I had a lot of people saying they could 'cure' me, and people visiting with weird and wonderful 'cures', from massaging my feet, massaging my head, tapping, pendants, all of which I smiled sweetly at. I tried using crystals – none of which worked, all of which were a complete and utter waste of time. And people were really misunderstanding what was going on, because a lot of these 'cures' misunderstood that if you did have some damage to your cells, your muscles, then tapping or massage to your feet was not going to stop or reverse the damage.*

I think a lot of them were as bad as the Health Protection Agency who said, it can't happen. People who said, if you think positively, it will be okay, you can fend it off. Well I'm afraid a little bit like smoking and asbestos, positive thinking can't stop the damage that cigarettes or tobacco can do to you, and it can't stop the damage that asbestos can do to you. I'm sure positive thinking is all very good – but, and a big but – it can't reverse what nature is doing to you.

I had become permanently more sensitive, although over time I recovered due to strict avoidance. I was having to turn the electricity off at night, it was giving me discomfort, so I decided as this was causing problems with the household, the fridge defrosting etc, to build an extension into the roof of the garage which allowed me to shield the whole of the room and have a separate electricity supply into the bedroom, so that at night when I went to bed not only was the room shielded against the masts around me – one mast at the front and one at the back – I was also able to turn the electricity off and that gave me some help.

I've certainly encouraged people to try and do this when they are living next door to people using Wi-Fi or a mast near their house.

The shield's made of layers of tin foil and metallised glass. This prevents the microwaves from masts from entering the bedroom.

I started to live a very restricted lifestyle – electricity off at night, keeping away from the TV, keeping away from the computer – I put them into one room in the house well away from the kitchen so that my wife could use those things and I could keep well away from them. Going to the theatre and the cinema became very difficult, but not impossible. Long haul flights where there were TVs etc in the aeroplane were a problem although short haul flights were fine, and the electronics from the cockpit and the engines were fine, it was the in-flight entertainment that caused me a problem.

During 2005, the UK Health Protection Agency began to conduct research to try to prove or disprove the condition of electrical sensitivity. Brian Stein was contacted by Dr James Rubin of the Psychology Department at King's College London.

I went down to see him to discuss taking part in the trials that he was designing. In the interview I suppose I became quite frightened at what he was asking people to do. You would have to put a mobile phone that was switched on to your head on a number of occasions. I explained to him that people who are electrically sensitive won't do that. That's a bit like saying to somebody with a peanut allergy, we'd like you to eat a jar of peanuts. That's okay, isn't it? No, it's not okay.

I was concerned that when I went to his office, I walked into the lobby area, and one door said ES Studies and another door said Gulf War Syndrome Studies. These were not scientists, they were psychologists. That made me worried and a little bit nervous. After being told how the study would take place, I backed out. That was not the correct way to treat people with electrical sensitivity. It was disrespectful and it would eliminate those people who were severely electrically sensitive. The best people who could prove this, would not do it. In conversations with the electrically sensitive community, all of them refused to take part in it. One, they didn't trust him, and two, they weren't going to put a mobile phone to their heads.

But shortly after that I had a communication from Essex University. They had a slightly different test, they were going to put people into a room, a Faraday Cage, where there would be a mast that was on or off. That sounded to me a bit more sensible, less damaging. So again I communicated with them and was happy to take part.

Brian Stein's Diary, The Essex Trials

I attended Essex University to discuss taking part in their ES trials in May, 2005. The two scientists conducting the trials were both psychologists and not physicists or biologists. This concerned me: was the research going to have a psychological slant?

They explained how the trial would be conducted. A series of medical questions, and then a thirty minute period in a Faraday cage with a hidden mast in the room, switched on and off for ten minute periods, double blind. Then at seven day intervals, fifty minute periods in the Faraday cage with the mast on for two occasions and off for one occasion, double blind.

I had a few questions. What was the strength of the mast? They didn't know. What screening procedure had been used to ensure that the people taking part were genuinely ES? None. 'Anyone who claimed they were ES could take part in the test,' they said. Had they discussed these individuals with any ES organisations to ensure they were sensible subjects? No.

My concern was that the results would be dependent on a very small group of people. If any frivolous individuals with a vested interest in the results could take part, they could easily be distorted. Their answers did not reassure me that they were taking this seriously. They appeared either naïve or had already made up their minds what the results would be, and that individuals could not be harmed by this test.

I asked this vetting question because not long before I had been asked by a friend to visit someone who claimed to be ES and help her. When I visited her it was clear that she had medical problems but she was not ES. She did however explain to me that she had signed up for the Essex trials to test if she was ES!

People like this would need to be vetted and removed – there was no procedure for doing so.

I asked why the mast was on twice and off once. Could it not be the other way around? The statistical significance of being correct was still the same, but someone who was made ill by being subjected to a mast for fifty minutes would successfully be able to continue, while someone who had to continue knowing they might be damaged again would have to pull out.

They told me: 'This is the test, take it or leave it.'

I asked if I was injured by the test, would I be ignored? They assured me this would not be the case. Even if I had to pull out early, my results would not be ignored?

I therefore after some trepidation signed up for the tests and started the short thirty minute experiments that day.

I explained that I would not be able to identify if a mast was on for ten minutes and then off for ten minutes and then on again for ten minutes. For most ES people it did not work like that. They would know if they had been exposed but they would not be able to pinpoint the time the exposure started. It was not like flicking a switch. A little like suffering from hay fever and being exposed to a freshly-cut field, if you were taken away from the pollen your hay fever did not stop, it continued for a long time afterwards. So it was with exposure to EMFs.

'That's the test, take it or leave it. You need to do this before the following fifty minute tests.'

I did the short exposure period, explained I could not pinpoint the time it was turned on or off, and was allowed to travel home.

I was at least reassured I would manage the exposure. I had been exposed to the signal for twenty minutes, and therefore, I thought, a fifty minute exposure should be okay.

How wrong could I be.

I returned to the University a week later, on the 18th of May, to be exposed this time for a fifty minute period (or not) in the double blind test.

During the fifty minute 'exposure' you took part in tests to check on the effectiveness of your brain. Simple recognition and memory tests: I thought this was worthless, because again they did not understand the association between exposure and after-effects. Although EMFs seriously affect the working of your brain, particularly in ES people, again it is not like flicking a switch. The effects are not felt immediately by most people, but over a period of time, which was too difficult to incorporate into the test: so you were checked during the exposure, which I knew would have limited value.

At the end of the fifty minutes they checked a few medical values, such as heart rate, blood pressure etc, and then asked whether I thought the mast had been off or on, and with what level of certainty. I explained that I was 60-70% certain that the mast had been on, but I would know better in a few hours' time when my body would react more if the mast had been on. They gave me a diary to be completed of the after-effects to be recorded over the next hours and the next seven days. I thought this was very relevant. I then disappeared to the lavatory before starting my journey home. They had given me directions to the lavatory and I found it, but on my return I got lost.

My internal navigation system is usually very good. I have noticed that when I have been exposed to EMFs I lose much of this innate ability. I was increasingly certain that the mast had been on – I was beginning to feel the effects.

On my journey home, which took 2.5 to 3 hours, I became more and more certain. The usual symptoms started to appear and by the time I reached home they had become more extreme than I had ever experienced. My bowels/stomach were in serious discomfort and on going to the lavatory it filled with blood. My stool was full of blood – not just a trace, but significant quantities. When I woke the following day, as well as still having blood in my stool, my brain was a fog: confused, disorientated, forgetful; some I had previously experienced after EMF exposure, but not to this extent.

I was frightened and concerned that I had done myself permanent damage. My brain remained in this fog for three days: when I woke on the fourth the fog had lifted and it was working normally again.

I also experienced discomfort in my chest, which was new. I had difficulty taking a deep breath and there was a new sensation deep inside. These sensations were difficult to describe, but unusual. Activity, pressure! All this was recorded in the diary given to me by the University and sent back to them by recorded delivery. I also telephoned to explain what had happened to me and that I would have to pull out of further testing. I was too frightened to be exposed to a further fifty minutes of EMFs: this was why I had wanted the mast to be on once, and off twice, because if this had been so, I was confident I would be able to go back and complete the trials.

The Essex Trials were commissioned by the UK Health Protection Agency and funded by the mobile phone industry.

*

Elsewhere, a community in Britain had taken matters into its own hands.

'The Future is Brighter Without Orange'

'ORANGE SQUASHED BY MAST ACTION WOMEN'

'Monday, October 24, 2005'

'Press Release - 24th October 2005'

'Mast Action UK'

'Orange Squashed by Mast Action Women'

'Today marks the end of a decade of campaigning against telecoms giant Orange.'

'At 8am today (24th October), Orange began dismantling the controversial mobile base station mast in Goffs Oak J.M.I. and Nursery School, which was erected in November 1995 under cover of night and without consultation with parents or local residents.'

'Christine Mangat and Julie Matthew, co-founders of the National Campaign Group Mast Action U.K., have won a landmark victory in their ten year struggle against corporate domination of the formulation and implementation of public policy:'

"We have maintained unremitting pressure on the MOA, Central Government (to bring the industry under tighter regulation) and Herts County Council, Broxbourne Borough Council and Goffs Oak JMI & Nursery School in our absolute determination to secure a safer environment for both school children and local residents. We have, at last, prevailed."

"Our future is brighter without Orange."

*

In the USA, the IEEE under C.K Chou succeeded in relaxing the safety levels for cell phones, the numbers of which were proliferating at a remarkable rate.

In Switzerland, the Swiss Agency for the Environment, Forests and Landscape (SAEFL) produced a booklet for every citizen entitled *'Electrosmog in the Environment.'*

The booklet explained the electromagnetic spectrum and addressed the issue of electrosmog and health, the 2000 Ordinance relation to non-ionising radiation, the impact of power lines and power stations, electrical appliances in the home, magnetic fields along railway lines, mobile telephony, broadcasting and amateur radio and wireless devices in buildings, including cordless phones, baby monitors and Wi-Fi:

'This brochure also addresses the aspect of personal responsibility – for electrosmog is often home-made. In many homes, the main sources of non-ionising radiation are not external supply systems, but rather our own electrical appliances.'

'And here, state legislation has its limitations in protecting us. It is therefore up to each of us to act in our own interest and make careful use of the many options provided by modern-day technology.'

'With a hands-free device, the distance from the antenna of the mobile phone is increased, and this reduces the level of radiation that can enter the head. To protect other sensitive parts of the body, when using a hands-free device the mobile phone should not be kept in a pocket near the heart or in a front trouser pocket.'

'The shorter the call using a mobile phone, the lower the exposure.'

'More and more wireless applications are now also being used indoors, e.g cordless phones, wireless headphones, baby monitors and WLAN stations for wireless connection to the Internet. Although their transmission power is often relatively low, these devices can dominate the indoor exposure to high-frequency radiation. To keep exposure as low as possible, these devices should be used at a due distance from places where people spend lengthy periods of time, including bedrooms, living rooms, home offices and children's rooms.'

'Baby monitors… Regardless of the type of device, wireless monitors should be kept at a minimum distance of 1.5 to 2 metres from the baby.'

The booklet would be imported into the UK in small numbers in the absence of any comparable initiative by the British government. Fifteen years on from publication, there was still no comparable initiative available to every citizen in Britain.

Brian Stein's Diary, 6 January 2006

I met up with Patricia Hewitt who was the Health Secretary and an MP in Leicester to discuss electrical sensitivity. She claimed she didn't know anything about it but during the course of the conversation it became clear that she did know all about Sweden, and Sweden accepting that electrical sensitivity did exist. She was very polite but not really interested in pursuing it. I had my meter with me and she asked me to scan her office to see if it was okay, and it was.

She made an interesting comment about Sir William Stewart: 'He's always telling us to take a precautionary approach' – as if this was a bloody nuisance.

So although the former head of the UK Health Protection Agency was saying, take a precautionary approach, the Health Secretary was not inclined to do so.

Later on that month I went to Wales, where a number of electrically sensitive people had arranged to have a week together. A number of these people were both electrically and chemically sensitive. Although I went there feeling sorry for myself, I came away feeling comparatively relieved, because for the people who were electrically and chemically sensitive it truly was a nightmare. Compared with them, I was relatively unaffected.

*

In Germany, *Hamburg Morgernpost* asked: 'Are We Telephoning Ourselves to Death?' In Denmark, *Dagens Medecin* declared: 'Mobile Phones Affect the Brain's Metabolism.'

In Sweden, a 'super' Wi-Fi system called WiMAX was installed as a blind test near the village of Gotene. The villagers were affected by headaches, blurred vision and heart arrhythmias. The moment the transmissions ceased, the symptoms disappeared.

Brian Stein's Diary, 2006

During March the results of the Essex University ES trials were published and there was no proof of electrical sensitivity. 60% of the people had recognised correctly that it (the mobile phone) was on, but it was not statistically significant. Therefore there was no proof.

On 28 July I spoke to Nigel Chilton from the UK Health Protection Agency in Cridland, near Didcot, and he was responsible for the MTHR programme on hypersensitivity studies. I explained to him what had happened to me at the Essex study, and I offered my services. I said that now I had recovered from taking part I was prepared to go back into the Faraday cage as many times as he wanted – 20, 50, 100 – and I would tell them on the one occasion when it was on – as long as it was off for all the others.

He declined, he said he couldn't do that, I was not statistically significant, and if the effects on me like blood in my stool were that dramatic, he wouldn't be able to get it through the ethics committee. So it would be 'unethical' to test me. But sadly not unethical to put a mobile phone mast near my house.

On 16 September, Stein travelled to Oxford to help man a stand at the university for a weekend show of charities and lectures on alternative medicine.

I noticed that it was a community that all got on with each other, they'd all been to other events before, and the only stand they kept away from was ours, which was talking about mobile phones and the damage they could do to you. Whether it was Save the Whale or Greenpeace or whatever, all these people spent the whole day on their mobile phones.

Of the people who did come to our stand, I would say there about single figures – 3-5% - we had a little chat with them and it was clear that that small percentage of people had a problem with their mobile phones. They were aware of it, it caused them discomfort.

So I would suggest there is a small percentage – 3-5% - who know there is an issue. That something is not right.

On 8 November I attended a Radiation Research Trust trustees meeting. Dr Ian Gibson, one of our trustees, said the only way the government will change its attitude is if there are bodies in the streets. The cabinet is not interested. Very depressing but probably very accurate.

Article in the Times from Nigel Hawkes, the health editor – 'Until somebody started the alarm over mobile phones, nobody except the mentally disturbed gave radio waves a second thought. It would be much better if these scares could be strangled at birth before they have a chance to become embodied in the psyche of the anxious.'

*

In December, a Danish mobile industry-sponsored study claimed to show little or no increase in cancers from mobile phone use and generated newspaper headlines such as *'Cell phones don't cause brain cancer'*. The study was criticised for its flawed methodology: it ignored cordless phones, mixed heavy and modest users in its data and was unable to persuade contract suppliers to heavy users to contribute to the study. Its subsequent publication in the *British Medical Journal* brought renewed criticism of the BMJ's editorial and peer review processes.

A response to this criticism also posted on the BMJ website declared: *'How many studies do we need to do to confirm that an exposure, for which there is no plausible mechanism of harm, does not actually do any harm? We need not waste any more public money on this.'* The response reputedly came from within the UK Health Protection Agency.

Brian Stein's Diary, 5 January, 2007

I received my results from the Essex studies. It showed that on the one day I attended where I was affected I was correct, the mast had been on. But as a result of not completing the tests my results will be ignored.

Brian Stein wrote back, and received a reply. The letter was again from Professor Elaine Fox of the Department of Psychology at Essex University: as he had completed only one of the three double-blind sessions, they were unable to use that data, including his follow-up questionnaire input, 'as we have nothing to compare it to.'

In the same week, Martin Anderson my sales director had a fit at work and was taken into hospital. He was diagnosed with a brain tumour. He's about 47, two young kids, mobile phone user. Sadly when he's communicated with me post the event he's on his mobile. He knows of my condition but it obviously doesn't have a great deal of effect on people.

I've lost any hope I had from the UK Health Protection Agency – these people are useless. I need to try and get another article in the paper, so I met up with a lady called Barbara Lantin on 24 January with a view to her doing an article for the Daily Mail.

Went for dinner at Langar Hall in Nottingham on 12 February. Frequently go there but this is the first time I've felt uncomfortable, something not quite right. Sure enough, they've installed Wi-Fi. I rang them and asked if it would be possible to turn it off in future when I was there, and got a pretty frosty response. So I need to start looking for somewhere other than Langar Hall to visit, which is a bit of a shame. It's the best restaurant in Nottinghamshire.

*

In February, 2007, Brian Stein continued his media campaign in the piece by Barbara Lantin in the *Daily Mail*:

'Can radiation from stereos, computers and other electric gadgets ruin your health? The experts say no, but this businessman's extraordinary story could force them to think again.'

The *Daily Mail* piece, unlike some newspapers when dealing with electrosensitive people, did not portray Stein as 'a freak', or an electro-refugee with a pony tail and a penchant for healing pendants who lived in a tepee. The newspaper gave him coverage as a successful business executive with status and credibility, who had a very real, yet barely recognised problem.

The article also cited Professor Olle Johansson of the Karolinska Institute in Stockholm, the Swiss study, and Professor Lawrie Challis, chairman of the Mobile Telecommunications and Health Research Programme, funded by the UK Government and the mobile 'phone industry, yet somehow 'independent of both.'

The MTHRP had just spent five years researching the 'short-term' effects of mobile phones and wireless masts: 'These are high quality studies' said Challis, 'and the signs are that they do not show any short-term effects from exposure to mobile phones.'

'What we have found is that when extra sensitive people are placed in conditions where they do not know whether a mobile phone is on or off, they are unable to tell more often than you would expect.'

Challis's 'short term' assertion was at odds with Brian Stein's experiences in the 24 hours and more after the Essex Trials.

'This needs further investigation,' Challis went on, 'Cancer takes more than ten years to appear: we have seen that with cigarettes, asbestos and the atomic bomb… We have no evidence so far of harm coming from mobile phones, but that does not mean that there is no harm… Short-term experiments do not tell us much about long-term effects. The only sure way of finding out whether there are long-term effects is to study people's health over a long period.'

Brian Stein was given the last word: 'I don't doubt my sanity, but I am concerned about the sanity of the rest of the world,' he had told the *Daily Mail*, 'Scientists used to say the earth was flat. I have no doubt that I will eventually be proved right.'

Brian Stein's Diary, 2007

The article in the Daily Mail appears on 20 February. Got telephone calls from 5Live, like to do an interview which I did, and interestingly I got a call the day of the article going in the press from Imogen at Langar Hall, apologising, and of course they will turn off the Wi-Fi for me, they hadn't realised, she was very nice! The Daily Mail did me a favour. I can still visit the best restaurant in Nottinghamshire.

Had a call from 5Live, they want to do live interview, half an hour, so I went down to London. They let me speak for about 30 seconds and it was a complete and utter waste of time. If I have half an hour I think I can convince people there's a problem – 30 seconds and it's just a joke.

On 21 February I met up with George Carlo. He's a gentleman from America who did some of the research into microwaves and discovered there was a problem. His theory is that 'information-carrying radio waves are detected by protein receptors in the cell membrane foreign invader response which closes down active transport channels interrupting gap junction communication and microbial flow preventing nutrients getting in and free radicals to escape resulting in apectosis cell suicide'... Phew!

Also at our meeting with the RRT we met a journalist from Panorama who was interested in doing a programme probably slanted towards Wi-Fi and schools.

The following day I had a meeting with George Carlo and Sir William Stewart at the HPA. His number two John Stathes was with him and Lawrie Challis. Sir William was interested in my story having read the article in the Daily Mail and wanted to know more. He seemed genuinely concerned and asked me if I would get involved in the design of the next studies.

After that meeting George Carlo and I had a meeting with Challis – Carlo and he did not see eye to eye at all – but it was also obvious to me that Challis would not allow me to get involved with any studies at all. He was very anti and seemed disparaging towards Sir William Stewart.

Following the Mail I had a number of radio interviews. What is interesting is the interviews you end up doing in the UK allow you a 30 second sound bite – then someone from the HPA comes in after you and rubbishes what you have just said. But on the 27th on Irish radio and the 28th on English speaking Spanish radio these people allow you half an hour. And you actually have a debate. And it's obvious during the course of the debate that they have become much more interested in what you are saying. It's not a 30 second pooh-poohing of the idea. They are happy to get engaged. But not in the UK.

Had a film crew arrive at my house from Richard and Judy. They said it would be 20-25 minutes in the show. I took part but the actual programme was 6 or 7 minutes – they claimed someone had pulled out which I would have thought would give us more time, but no, they had to put a pre-recorded session in, which meant we had less time, and the result was it was a bit of a joke, it was not treated seriously.

I had two and half minutes to talk and that was it. The representative from the industry was a nuclear physicist who admitted to me he knew nothing at all about non-ionising radiation.

I was told by the crew after the event that the UK Health Protection Agency was due to attend, but they (the HPA) wanted to know who was going to be on. When my name was mentioned they refused to put anyone on the programme.

Katie Morgan from the BBC confirmed the Panorama team would be doing a programme on Wi-Fi and masts. She will be interviewing some of the WHO scientists and Sir William Stewart.

In April, 2007, the warnings and recommendations of the 2000 Ecolog Study (**see link in Appendix 5**) commissioned and buried by T-Mobil in Germany were leaked to the Human Ecological

Social Economic Project and thence to the media. Seven years on, the mobile phone industry had significantly increased its 'war-gaming' and counterpropaganda, and in spite of their implications the revelations concerning the Ecolog Study findings aroused little coverage.

Brian Stein's Diary, 2007

Had a meeting at Sainsburys with Mike Coupe and a number of suppliers on the directors' floor. Opposite there was a bank of masts on the roof of the building next door, which is as close as I have ever been at a working position to a mast. This affected me badly. All these masts are irradiating the 7th floor of Sainsburys head office. It will be fascinating to see how many directors and people who work for the directors of Sainsburys on the 7th floor get affected by masts in the coming years.

Meanwhile continuing to bleed when I am exposed to Wi-Fi or masts or a bit too much EMFs. Started to have a conversation – insisted on by my wife – with the doctor. Having a colonoscopy to see if there are any problems but treated quite badly by the doctors when you say you are ES. They don't take it terribly seriously.

8 May, 2007: Had my second colonoscopy. Quite polite but don't think they believe a word of it when you explain you are ES and why you are bleeding. Told me there was no reason, all okay, nothing to worry about.

Meanwhile I continue to bleed when I'm in a Wi-Fi environment.

The government have got wind of the Panorama programme Sir William Stewart is appearing on and are not very happy. Sir William Stewart is not very happy that they have found out about it. On 21 May the programme goes out – it will be interesting to see what the reaction will be. I think Sir William Stewart has been quite brave. Let's see what happens.

*

On 20 May, 2007, the BBC screened the Panorama programme 'Wi-Fi: the Warning Signals', which featured interviews with Sir William Stewart, author of the Stewart Report and Head of the UK Health Protection Agency, Professor Olle Johansson of the Karolinska Institute in Stockholm, Dr Gerd Oberfeld, who had highlighted the possible biological effects of wireless microwaves in schools in Austria, Alasdair Philips of Powerwatch, Philip Parkin, General Secretary of the Professional Association of Teachers, who expressed concern at the quantity of Wi-Fi in school rooms, and Dr Michael Repacholi, head of the World Health Organisation research programme into radio frequency radiation and founder of ICNIRP - upholders of the mobile phone industry's 'no adverse health effects' school of thinking.

Repacholi, who had reputedly helped unseat Gro Harlem Brundtland as the head of the WHO after she publicly revealed her electrosensitivity and misgivings about mobile phones, was probably the most powerful person featured in the programme. He gave a robust defence of the industry's position. As Brian Stein noted in his diary:

The comment post-Panorama was 'It's scaremongering.' The fact that it was Sir William Stewart saying these things, it was as if it was a lobby of lunatics talking, not the head of the Health Protection Agency.

But there was more to come from a mobile phone industry increasingly sensitive about any questioning of its practices in the mainstream media.

Meanwhile in Sidney, Australia, a retired telecom worker hijacked a tank and rammed six microwave towers to the ground. In Galilee, Israel, a Druze community protested at the erection of a new microwave tower on the grounds that the towers already there had caused rising rates of cancer. The tower was built, but soon afterwards local teenagers burned it down. When the police arrived, the Druze rioted, injuring more than twenty-five officers.

The European Environment Agency warned that *'cell phone technology could lead to a health crisis similar to those caused by asbestos, smoking and lead in petrol.'*

Brian Stein's Diary, 25 July 2007

Went up to Tulken (in Scotland) with Samworth Brothers. Although everything very low tech noticed a problem in the house, very uncomfortable for an hour or so, then started going round the house to find out what could be causing it. Sure enough, they've got detectors plugged into the mains to frighten mice. I unplugged them and I was fine.

Whilst in Tulken the results of the Essex study were released. Surprise, surprise, it's all in the mind. I was contacted by the BBC and the Independent. The BBC wanted an interview. I explained what had happened to me and the bleeding etc and they made something of it for a day or so.

Meanwhile life becomes even more inconvenient. Coming back from the Midlands in the summer I managed to get involved in the floods and it took me 12 hours to get home, so by that time even my little Micra was affecting me. So all cars now affect me and I am having to limit my use of a car and get driven around much of the time, either by my wife or by a friend to work. Life becomes even more difficult.

Scepticism was growing among the ES community about the methodology and findings – *'Study finds health symptoms aren't linked to mast emissions'* - of the Essex Trials.

Brian Stein's Diary, 2007

In October the government announce they are going to do some research into Wi-Fi. We've made some suggestions as to how they might do that. Typical government, doing research into what they already know the answer to. They are going to check if the levels of Wi-Fi in schools are above or below the ICNIRP levels. There's no need to spend money doing that because we already know they'll be well below the ICNIRP levels.

On 26 November attended a conference in London 'Human Health in an Electro-Technological World' at the Royal Society organised by Roger Coghill. Met Roger Coghill, Olle Johansson, John Walker, Chris Busby, Lennart Hardell. On the 27th Cindy Sage presented the research from the Bioinitiative Review. She and Lennart Hardell very impressive and knowledgeable on the subject and the science.

*

On 30 November, 2007, the BBC upheld complaints against Panorama's '*WiFi: the Warning Signals*' that the programme 'gave a misleading impression of the state of scientific opinion on the issue' and suggested following a complaint from Michael Repacholi that his evidence 'was presented in a context which suggested to viewers that his scientific independence was in question, whereas the other scientists were presented uncritically.' As Brian Stein observed in his diary: *'The BBC have been got at.'*

Brian Stein's Diary, 2007

Lots of politics with ES-UK. The secretary has been removed, probably a good thing if we are going to make the organisation professional. I'm one of the people getting the blame. Then all of a sudden, rumours circulating, 'Brian Stein's friendly with the mobile phone industry and he's a plant'. Sadly this is what happens whenever you upset some people from the ES community. They can be quite nasty!

I also had a letter from Professor Elaine Fox at Essex University. She wanted to discuss the results of my study with the press and she needs a disclaimer from me to allow this to happen. I rang her and the conversation went something along the lines, she wants me to sign a disclaimer, I am very happy to do so as long as they discuss all of my results, the only results she wants to discuss with the press are the first day, when I said I couldn't tell any difference, and not the following week's one hour test because I didn't complete that.

I said the only way I would allow them to discuss my texts would be if they discussed all the tests I did, including the follow up papers I sent about my internal bleeding. What follow up papers, she asked? I explained that the university gave us follow up papers to fill in over the next hours and days. She didn't know anything about them. Which is very sad, because that was probably the most important information of all.

Bizarre. I explained to her that I bled internally after taking part in the test – which she told me was impossible. I queried how could she possibly say this, when I was taking part in the test. Had she already decided that it was impossible? She then hung up on me.

These people should be held to account in the years to come.

Brian Stein's Diary, 2008

Research from Gerd Oberfeld in Austria showing 850% increase in cancers within 200 metres of a mast. This was challenged by the mobile phone industry and they're threatening to sue him because they are claiming the mast in question has never been turned on. Why they would put up a mast and not turn it on, not too sure. He doesn't have the resources to take on the mobile phone industry and I think he might have to back down. The records of the mast never being turned on have been lost – so no proof, simply the word of the mobile phone operator! (NB Austrian mobile phone operators have subsequently been required by law to keep these records.)

*

The Interphone Study involving 13 countries (but not the US) by International Agency for Research on Cancer, Lyon, France, reported that, after a decade of mobile phone use, the chances of getting developing a brain tumour on the side of the head where the phone was used went up as much as 40% for adults.

Brian Stein's Diary, April 14 2008

Meeting at Westminster with Andrew Mitchell MP and Stewart Eke from the Mobile Phone Operators Association (MPOA). I think Andrew is prepared to ask a few awkward questions in the presence of the MPOA, but then not really prepared to take it further. A lot of platitudes, anybody who's an MP has got to think about the economy, and they're not prepared to push this area too hard.

The National Library of France announced it was shutting down its Wi-Fi system, and the Library of Sainte-Genevieve called for the replacement of its Wi-Fi networks with hard-wired connections. *The Age* (Australia) headlined '*Scientists Warn of Mobile Phone Cancer Risk.*'

In the same month, the EM Radiation Research Trust held its first conference on the Global issue of EMF and Health, 8-9 September, Royal Society, London. The strapline ran: 'This Conference is about resolution not revolution.'

A *Who's Who* of the wireless world attended – Sir William Stewart, Dr Henry Lai, Michael Repacholi, Professor Lennart Hardell, Professor Olle Johansson, Professor Yury Grigoriev, Paolo Vecchia, George Carlo, Cindy Sage, Dr Ulrich Warnke, James Rubin, Gerd Oberfeld, Grahame Blackwell, MPs including Joe Benton, Ian Gibson, Phil Willis and Andrew Mitchell, Green MEPs including Caroline Lucas, Senator Mark Daly, and ES-UK and RRT supporters and trustees including Brian Stein and Eileen O'Connor:

'This is the first time that the leaders from both sides - 'there is no problem' and 'we have a serious problem'- have been brought together for such a debate.' The UK Health Protection Agency pulled out at the last moment – Sir William Stewart stepped in to keep it on track.

Brian Stein's Diary, 8 September 2008

The RRT conference. Sadly not a great deal of interest from the press. Anything they do is one or two little soundbites. I made my speech but sadly the gentleman we engaged to do the recording has been filming all day and only found out at the end of the day that the sound has not been working!

In his speech, Professor Yury Grigoriev, deputy chairman of the Russian Non-Ionising Radiation Protection Federation, announced that they had 100 years' research proving that EMFs cause cancer.

On challenging Mike Repacholi from ICNIRP as to whether or not this research was reviewed by ICNIRP, Repacholi explained that this research was published in Russian and therefore ignored. Only research published in English was reviewed. Russia's EMF levels are significantly below that allowed in the UK.

The Sage Report was presented showing the thousands of research papers documenting damage from EMFs. The mobile phone industry audience nitpicked at the report. They regard all scientists who find damage from EMFs as campaigners and not scientists. They have a very powerful lobby and are very intimidating. I can understand why researchers are loath to do research finding damage from EMFs.

Dinner in the evening at the House of Commons. All the speakers were very impressed. Sat next to David Coggan who was obviously very anti and quite awkward with being placed next to me.

Day 2, the mobile phone industry very hostile. We thought we could bring the two sides together, but that's very naïve. I don't see how we can make inroads in bringing them together until there are enough people who are dying.

Mike Repacholi mentioned at the conference that he thought the Radiation Research Trust could have some input into one of the ICNIRP subcommittees but nothing ever happened about it.

A little bit of publicity from one or two papers – the Sunday Independent – but absolutely nothing at all in the Times or the Guardian.

Brian Stein's Diary, 2009

Eileen O'Connor and I go to a conference in Brussels in advance of the EC debating the issue next week. I sense the European scientists are very complacent and smug.

The second day of the conference was much better. A number of comments were made by members of the audience who were ES and this seemed to influence some of the European legislators and rattle the mobile phone operators. There was also a scientist from the Karolinska Institute who was very very anti, and claimed that Sweden doesn't recognise ES. They recognise that some people are ill, a bit like the UK, but it has nothing to do with EMFs.

During the course of the debate, what was fascinating was that the executive clearly stated they take their advice from ICNIRP. So they simply comply and if there's a problem it's not their fault. Then the mobile phone operators say they are following the rules that are laid down by the executive and ICNIRP. So if there's a problem, it's not their fault. Health and safety is not their responsibility, it is ICNIRP and the executive's responsibility.

Then when ICNIRP spoke they said that they were giving guidance on the results, the thermal effects, of known science. The standards relate to the thermal effects and it is up to the executive to interpret their advice. So, if it is biological effects that cause the problem, then it's not their fault, it's down to individual countries to leigislate for chronic non-thermal effects.

So clearly no-one is accepting any responsibility. If there's a problem in the future, it's not their fault.

It sounds a bit like the banking crisis.

On 28 March, 2009, I went to see my MP, Ken Clarke. I explained to him that I was electrically sensitive and I had some research that I would like him to look at. He immediately went on the attack. I was a trouble maker. I was a conspiracy theorist. There was no danger with mobile phones. He refused to take or read any of the literature that I had. And he terminated the meeting with those comments!

This is was our Justice Minister.

28 May, 2009: Met John Quinn, Prof of Neurobiology at the University of Liverpool. Again no matter how much you tell these scientists, they simply don't believe you. He was aware of the debate, was very polite but really did not want to get involved.

24 June, 2009: Had a letter from the cancer screening programme. Another abnormal result, they found blood in my stool. Now there's a surprise! Is it worth going for any more check ups with them the way they treat me? I don't know.

Looking to purchase a holiday home in Cornwall or Devon away from masts and radar. One would think that this would be easy to do. It's a nightmare trying to find a house that is not within a couple of miles of a mast. It's not easy. Likewise going on holiday to a new location is difficult. Hotels without Wi-Fi are getting harder to find.

Involved in the publication of the 15 Reasons document why they are underscoring the possibility of brain tumours. Caused quite a sensation over in America. Lots of TV and radio interviews in the US. All very quiet in the UK.

An independent study in Sweden reported that people who had started using a mobile phone before the age of 20 were five times more likely to develop a brain tumour. The Austrian Medical Association called for a ban on Wi-Fi in schools, citing children's thinner skulls and the danger to their nervous systems. Austrian and other insurers also decided not to indemnify mobile phone companies against health claims by users.

By 2009, the number of cell phone antennae in the US had risen from 19,850 in 1995 to 247,000, most of them featuring multiple antennae. Fees paid for frequency portions had risen from US $8 billion in 1996 to US $52 billion.

In the USA, Dr Samuel Milham's paper was published: *'Most cancer in firefighters is due to radio-frequency radiation exposure not inhaled carcinogens.'*

'Recent reviews and reports of cancer incidence and mortality in firefighters conclude that they are at an increased risk from a number of cancers. These include leukaemia, multiple myeloma, non-Hodgkin's lymphoma, males breast cancer, malignant melanoma, and cancers of the brain, stomach, colon, rectum, prostate, urinary bladder, testes, and thyroid. Firefighters are exposed to a long list of recognized or probable carcinogens in combustion products and the presumed route of exposure to these carcinogens is by inhalation. Curiously, respiratory system cancers and diseases are usually not increased in firefighters as they are in workers exposed to known inhaled carcinogens. The list of cancers with increased risk in firefighters strongly overlaps the list of cancers at increased risk in workers exposed to electromagnetic fields (EMF) and radio frequency radiation (RFR)...'

'I suggest that some of the increased cancer risk in firefighters is caused by RFR exposure, and is therefore preventable. The precautionary principle should be applied to reduce the risk of cancer in firefighters, and workmen's compensation rules will necessarily need to be modified.'

Brian Stein's Diary, 3 October 2009

We had an ES-UK conference. Olle Johansson, Alasdair Phillips, Denis Henshaw, Anne Silk and Andrew Goldsworthy. Good speakers and good response from the audience. One hundred severely ES people attended.

The Open University are very good with disability students. They send me transcripts of the recordings I've got to listen to and I'm allowed to take my exams (BS is studying for a Law Degree) at home rather than in a Wi-Fi environment. I have an invigilator who comes to sit opposite me to make sure I don't cheat, but they do put themselves out for you.

15 November, 2009: Drove to Birmingham with Eileen to attend a conference in Norway. The idea was to get together with a group of scientists and concerned individuals from different associations to see if we can agree a way forward and set new standards – better than ICNIRP's – of what levels of emissions should be allowed.

Had a chat with the scientist who headed up the Reflex Project. The industry is simply throwing mud at any researchers who find there is a problem. And indeed throwing mud personally at him. He was a respected scientist until he found that microwaves damage DNA.

In the USA, journalist Christopher Ketcham called *Microwave News* founder Louis Slesin. Slesin had used the US Freedom of Information Act to access online many key but little-reported studies linking microwave radiation and increased risk of cancer, commissioned by or submitted to the Defense Department and the FDA:

'No-one in this country cared,' Slesin said of the Swedish findings, 'it wasn't news! We love our cell phones. The paradigm that there's no danger here is part of a worldview that had to be put into place. Americans are not asking the questions, maybe because they don't want the answers. So what will it take?'

Twenty-four years after the EPA halted his research, Carl Blackman told Ketcham: 'A decision was made to stop the civilian agencies from looking too deeply into the non-thermal health effects from exposure to EM fields. Scientists who have shown such effects over the years have been silenced, had funding taken away, been laughed at, been called charlatans and con men. The goal was to only let in scientists who would say, 'We know that microwave ovens can cook meat, and that's all we need to know.'

Another veteran EPA physicist, speaking anonymously, told Ketcham: 'The Department of Defense didn't like our research because the exposure limits that we might recommend would curtail their activities.'

Christopher Ketcham drove down to visit Allan Frey: 'If we had looked into it a little more,' Frey told him, 'if we had done the real science, we could have allocated spectrums that the body can't feel. The public should know if they are taking a risk with cell phones. What we're doing is a grand world experiment without informed consent.'

'Until there are bodies in the streets,' Frey said, 'I don't think anything is going to change… When it comes to this matter, the IEEE is a charade.' He also told Devra Davis that there was 'quite a history' of deliberately doctored (sic) trials in this field and that 'we are looking in the wrong places.' Then he sailed away on his boat – but presumably not out of reach of electromagnetic fields.

That December, in Italy, a landmark court decision awarded disability compensation to Innocenzo Marcolini, a business executive, on the grounds that his brain tumour was the result of non-thermal radiation from protracted mobile phone use. His employers appealed.

Brian Stein's Diary, 2010

In early January I start to notice I am bleeding more. I've been to see my doctor. Arranged another colonoscopy. It's almost as if they don't believe I'm bleeding.

11 January, 2010: RRT meeting. Oleg Grigoriev made a presentation. The Russians are now building shielded rooms in hospitals to treat and research electrical sensitivity. They seem to be light years ahead of us. They offered to present their research to the HPA. The HPA declined.

Met up with John Mann MP near North Whitley with Sue Ledgard (an ES sufferer). He put himself out, came to her house, had a long chat but basically I don't think he's interested in helping us. Too many other pressing issues.

Went on a skiing holiday with the kids. They managed to find a resort in France where they could turn the Wi-Fi off. It was wonderful: my first time skiing. One night I woke up at 3am trembling, terrible tinnitus, seriously agitated. Something was not right. Went downstairs and discovered that the kids had been watching TV last thing at night and without realising it they'd plugged in the Wi-Fi. It had been on since late at night and my system had recognised it. Who says it's psychosomatic?

There's an e-forum coming up at Westminster to discuss smart meters. I rang up and asked to speak and they said yes. Then I told them why, I didn't want them installed, and these were he reasons why, and all of a sudden the bookings had been made, the speakers were already arranged and they couldn't possibly have me speaking! Well there's a surprise!

I'm becoming slightly chemically sensitive as well and having known some people who were chemically sensitive that's a scary possibility. Hopefully I can control it.

*

In February, 2010, *GQ* Magazine published Christopher Ketcham's piece *'Warning: Your Cell Phone May Be Hazardous to Your Health'* regarding cell 'phone hazards in the USA.

In April, in Bangalore, India, new restrictions were introduced on the use of mobile phones by students and teachers. In Egypt, the Abdel-Rassoul study revealed sleep impairment and memory loss among people living close to wireless masts.

In the UK, the COSMOS long-term industry-funded project was announced into mobile phones and health hazards. The project would be dismissed as buying time for the industry by independent researchers and in the ES-UK 3/12 newsletter.

Brian Stein's Diary, 5 July, 2010

Presented at the Common Purpose group and had it filmed. Going to use that for setting up my Electromagneticman.co.uk website.

21 August, 2010: Went for colonoscopy with Mr Abercrombie, a new doctor. He was much more skilled at doing it. He found a polyp and removed it. The polyp was cancerous. And having removed it, all my bleeding has stopped. I asked him how long it takes to develop and he tells me about seven years – which is about the time I first started bleeding when I attended the Essex Trials.

27 October, 2010: Met up with Mr Abercrombie. He confirmed it was cancerous, not sure whether the surface of the polyp touching the colon was cancerous or not, but the cancer team are recommending that they remove one third of my colon. I'm not very keen on this. I explained that the hospital is not a good place for me to go into, is there an alternative? He explains that although the team are keen on removing it his personal advice is to leave it and monitor it. So we agree to see what happens, and as it happens the subsequent scans are clear as is another colonoscopy and he's happy that I'm clear of cancer and we'll leave it three years before we do another colonoscopy. So fingers crossed, I'm quite lucky, I've caught it just in time because of my own perseverance.

2 November, 2010: In London with Devra Davis. She's publicising her book. Met up with a journalist who questioned her and the journalist told me she got her advice about this area from Sense About Science which is a bit of a joke. You can sense the hostility towards Devra Davis from the UK Health Protection Agency and the scientific community. They are not very happy at all about her being given the opportunity to lecture to people in the UK.

Met up with Kevin O'Neill, brain surgeon. He's started to get involved with Mobilewise because he's seeing significant increases in brain tumours in the people he's treating, and while the government are saying there's a 0-2% increase in brain tumours, he's seeing a 15% increase.

19 November, 2010: The UK Health Protection Agency EMF and Health Teach-in. Looking at the printed notes they provided, they were very sensible, but listening to the scientists was slightly different. The spin that they put on when they spoke was disgraceful. Clarke said it made no sense to him at all, that people should be frightened about masts, 'common sense' told him they could not cause a problem. Someone else dismissed South American research into fertility as poorly carried out. I explained about my particular issue, and they didn't really want to know.

They did mention that children might be vulnerable. They did mention that SAR levels can exceed the ICNIRP guidelines with children, but they didn't think they needed to do anything about it. They discredited the Bioinitiatives Report because it was written by 'campaigning scientists' who were not 'real' scientists. They described the opposition as uneducated and unscientific and then Swerdlow did an assassination job on Lennart Hardell. He was an 'extreme' scientist who came up with 'extreme' results, they were not credible, not reliable.

I mentioned to him that US scientists had checked brain tumour results for rigor and that Lennart Hardell was the gold standard and some of the research he was quoting was coming out near the bottom. He simply ignored me. They had brainwashed people so well that somebody in the audience even said, why are we wasting our money on this research, there's no need to do any more research, it's perfectly safe, we should be doing research into diet and obesity. And all the scientists on the platform smiled and nodded in agreement.

Brian Stein's Diary, 4 April 2011

I had a request from Talk Sport to do an interview on ES which I agreed to do. I recorded this and it went out in the early hours of *the morning when nobody was listening to it. But interestingly enough the following day I had a message from James Russell, a film producer who had been driving home and listening to it. He's interested in doing a film about ES and the dangers of mobile phones. So it was worth doing it in the middle of the night!*

14 April, 2011: A visit from James Russell. He wants to start in May, targeting C4, he sounds like he's somebody who could make a difference.

In May, 2011, the World Health Organisation – from which Dr Gro Harlem Brundtland had been unseated eight years earlier as Director-General after she spoke publicly about the health hazards of mobile 'phones - in its Sheet 193 classified electromagnetic fields as a Class 2B carcinogen (comparable to lead and DDT).

The International Agency for Research on Cancer (IARC), based partly on work by Lennart Hardell and Interphone, reclassified electromagnetic fields as a 2B carcinogen: i.e possibly carcinogenic.

Brian Stein's Diary, 8 June 2011

RRT trustees meeting met Erica Mallery-Blythe, an emergency doctor who has been working in America although she's British. She's very impressive and very concerned about the effects of EMFs. We've asked her to become a trustee.

10 June, 2011: After the IARC reclassification the Australian centre for Radio Frequency Bioeffects have closed down their research because they have decided that EMFs are safe!

27 July, 2011: We started our 'Save the Male' campaign in loos dotted up and down the motorway services in the UK. We can only afford to have them in there for one week but hopefully we can stir up a debate.

Interestingly enough before the week is out we've had a message from the Advertising Standards Authority (ASA) who want us to remove them because they've had complaints. I wonder from whom?

We've actually had more publicity from the complaints than we have had from the campaign. BBC Radio Solent and other local radio stations.

The ASA want proof of sperm damage. We've responded to the Advertising Standards Authority saying that the Council of Europe has sent advice to member states that governments should warn populations of the danger of EMFs and withdraw Wi-Fi from areas where children are situated. Most of the research we've seen on fertility shows that EMFs damage it, and this is why we did the Save the Male campaign. 80% of peer research shows damage to sperm.

The eventual Advertising Standards Authority ruling was that the complainers were correct. It is not 'generally accepted' in the UK that EMFs damaged sperm, and therefore you can't warn people that it might!

August, 2011: Had the news of another of my directors: David Pilling has a brain tumour. He's not a big mobile phone user, but he has a cordless system at home and Wi-Fi. When he's ringing me to tell me he's recovering, he's on his cordless phone, and within a short period of time the tumour is back, and within a short period of time after that, David Pilling has died.

In August, 2011, *Scientific American* declared there was 'no threat'. However, in an Italian TV programme later that year it would be alleged that many scientists had expected the IARC grading to be Class 2A, and that in spite of ICNIRP apparently declaring the personal interest of each member, four people on IARC had potential conflicts of interest which were not disclosed at the time: Clemens Dasenbrock, Fraunhofer Institute, Germany, funded by the GSM Association and the Mobile Manufacturers Forum; Tomoyuki Shirai, Nagoya City University, retired, funded by the Association of Radio Industry and Business in Japan; Junji Miyakoshi, Kyoto University, Japan, funded by the same; and Juuka Jutilainen, University of Eastern Finland, funded by the GSM Association and the Mobile Manufacturers Forum.

On 24 September, 2011, the ES-UK Conference on Electrical Sensitivity was held at Melton Mowbray, Leicestershire. Dr Diana Samways was a retired General Practitioner from Haslemere in Surrey, with an interest in mould allergies:

I stayed 2 nights at a nearby hotel, and was introduced by the hotelier to a man (whom we'll call' X') who was going to the conference. We sat at the same table for breakfast.

'X' looked ill, pale puffy face, eyes like slits, and an air of discomfort and twitchiness. He wore (at all times) a high visibility fluorescent jacket with silver reflective stripes. I gave him a lift to the conference which was held in a lecture room with no electricity, no mobile phones etc. to cater for the visitors who were all electrically sensitive. (No lights, no projector, no visual aids.)

There were 100 people and the degree and diversity of disability was startling. Some in wheelchairs, one so allergic she couldn't go anywhere near the coffee machine and much else. Many had multiple allergies and multiple chemical sensitivity.

I sat near the door of the lecture room. There was a constant traffic of people going out (and in) because they felt too ill to listen, including my friend 'X' who went in and out very many times over the day (and fell down a step he failed to see.)

Dr Samways had witnessed many things in her career as a GP, but never anything like this: '*On thinking about this whole experience afterwards, I realised that I had stumbled into a very serious problem that the authorities are not acknowledging and GPs are not diagnosing correctly.*'

Two weeks after the ES-UK Conference, Dr Samways led a workshop on electrosensitivity at Bosham House Conference Centre. She told the story of the Conference:

Afterwards an attendee who was a senior sister at St James' psychiatric hospital down the road said they had four patients who had been certified and locked up as manic depressives who in her opinion were not so. They had been sectioned for 'bipolar disease' but they were not typical. Manic depressives are very happy with their mania, buying things with money they haven't got and running around the garden nude. Often very respectable people.

Normally these patients like their 'high' and feel good, whereas her four were very unhappy and twitchy on their 'high' and quite different. She also said they had past histories of heavy computer and/or mobile phone use (bankers.)

What she described sounded very like my observation of 'low level chaos.' I don't know what happened to these people, but suspect they were incarcerated and sedated. Hospitals are full of electrical equipment which would make them worse, not better, and the diagnosis was being missed. (I offered to lead a workshop for the nurses at this hospital, but have heard no more.)

*

In October, 2011, in the UK, the *Epping Forest Guardian* reported on headaches, dizzy spells, sleeplessness and nosebleeds experienced by residents since O2 and Vodafone built a 60 foot microwave mast near their homes.

In the same month, in the USA, ABC News carried a story about people who had moved to West Virginia to live in the 'quiet zone' around the large radio telescope. The quiet zone was free of Wi-Fi which would have interfered with the telescope's operation.

Also in the USA, *East County* magazine carried a piece by Lisa Rene Anderson, who had moved to Shelter Valley to escape the effects of EM radiation in San Diego, only to find that a telecom company had plans to install a 45 foot multi-antenna tower in the middle of the town.

She reiterated that Clinton's 1996 Federal Communications Act was based on false claims, and the fact that 45 cities in California had banned Wi-Fi smart meters and *'many parents are successfully working to keep Wi-Fi radiation out of their children's schools. It is time that our Planning Commissions in America take back their power from the 15 year-old Telecommunications Act that has hog-tied them for so long and resume their job of protecting our lives and environment.'*

In France, *Romandie News* reported that two women had taken refuge in a cave without heat or electricity in the Hautes-Alpes to escape microwave masts and Wi-Fi. Anne and Bernadette Cautain Touloumond were a former technical officer from a university in Nice and a former air hostess. The former, suffering from headaches, had previously slept in a car, a cellar restaurant, underground car parks and fields in Burgundy. The latter said: 'When I found myself in this cave, I could not believe it and wondered what I did to get here.' She had been called crazy, lost most of her friends and her family were baffled.

Brian Stein's Diary, 2011

James Rubin cites such newspaper reports as evidence that electrosensitivity is psychosomatic. He argues that these people who 'want to live in caves' are frightened of technology, and that such people have existed since time began. They are frightened of progress, frightened of anything new.

In my experience, most ES people are ES because they love the technology. They are ill because they have overused it. Most are ES and still trying to find ways to use the technology. It is only a very small percentage who become so sensitive that they resort to leaving their family and friends to go and live in a cave. Rubin is using hearsay and anecdotal evidence to make his point – while anecdotal evidence proving the opposite is ignored and not reported.

*

David Gee, Senior Advisor on science, policy and emerging issues at European Environment Agency, warned again in its Newsletter and called for precautionary measures regarding EMFs, citing the precedent of smoking and lung cancer, now accepted in spite of the fact that the biological mechanisms of the latter *are still not fully understood...The cost of these measures is very low, but the potential costs of inaction may be very high.'*

Brian Stein's Diary, 7 October, 2011

We had a reply from the Advertising Standards Authority upholding the complaint against 'Save The Male'. Surprise, surprise! Generally not accepted that EMFs cause fertility problems, so therefore we were wrong to publicise it. We explained how was it possible for a truth to become known if you weren't allowed to publicise it? Even with the Council of Europe saying that we should? But they ignored that and told us we weren't allowed to proceed.

The Man in the Silver Suit

In Sweden, the *Swedish Local* reported on Dan Bengtsson, who wore a silver suit to reduce the effects of electrosmog in central Sweden. Bengtsson and the local authority called for the redirection of masts and the creation of clear zones, to which the industry replied that this would make TV and mobile phones unworkable.

ES-UK campaigned against the arbitrary installation of domestic Wi-Fi 'smart' gas and electricity meters, citing the threat to health and the precedent of California and the successful fibre optic alternative in Italy. The specific issue raised the general profile of electrosensitivity and its sufferers.

Questions were asked in the UK House of Commons about 'smart' meters and the non-thermal threat from Wi-Fi. Customers would be able to opt out of having a smart meter installed: but what about the family living above or below?

In France, the ASEF Environmental Health Association reported on the effects of microwave masts on social housing residents in

Aix-en-Provence and Aubagne. Social housing tenants had no right to object to masts: the report showed high incidences of sleep disturbance, memory impairment and noise pollution – all of which disappeared when people went away on holiday.

In Brussels, the Electrosmog Protest took place at the EMF and Health Conference. As part of the accompanying literature, Olle Johansson wrote: *'There have been countless papers in scientific journals over several decades that show very clearly that there are non-thermal biological effects (some of them extremely harmful) of electromagnetic fields that are well below the official safety guidelines.'*

In November, 2011, in the USA, Christopher Ketcham's article 'Warning: High Frequency' in *Earth Island Journal* contained numerous accounts: the upstate New York sculptress whose life collapsed after a smart meter was installed, and who recovered to some degree after it was removed; the Los Alamos scientist threatened with dismissal after asking for protection from electromagnetic fields in his laboratory; the activist and former publisher of 'No Place to Hide' Arthur Firstenberg who now lived out of the back of his car in the wilderness; the former world record marathon runner who lived out of her car for eight years before settling in a house surrounded by mountains.

In the same month, in Washington, USA, the internationally respected scientist Henry Lai circulated a recently declassified USAF paper concerning the Soviet bombardment with microwaves of the US Embassy in Moscow during the Cold War.

The author Paul Brodeur in *'The Zapping of America'* had previously published detailed allegations surrounding the subject, including the secret testing by the US State Department of young women from the Moscow Embassy in the 1960s, where genetic damage was allegedly confirmed, and the fact that several US ambassadors to Moscow had died of cancer. National Security Advisor to President Carter, Zbigniew Brezinzinski, had also stated in 1978 that the cancer rate among Americans in the Moscow Embassy was 'the highest in the world.'

The declassified report circulated by Dr Lai prompted responses citing a 2012 paper on the matter by Mark Ellwood asserting the 'no adverse health effects' position in the case of the Moscow Embassy, noting that Mr Ellwood was working for the Cancer Research Trust (Dunedin) at the request of Telecom New Zealand, for whom Ellwood had prepared other reports.

The room, however, was against Ellwood – the term 'whitewash' was used – and with Dr Lai, Brodeur and John Goldsmith: the latter of whom in a highly-regarded study had reported *'elevated mutagenesis and carcinogenesis among the employees and dependents that were chronically exposed to a very low intensity radar signal at the US Embassy in Moscow from the 1950s to the 1970s.'*

Brian Stein's Diary, 13 December 2011

We met up with Patrick Mercer MP in London and went along to 10 Downing Street. Bill Esterson and Joe Benton MPs came along with us and presented a document on the dangers of wireless smart meters.

A number of EU countries including France and Germany have decided that all smart meters will be hard-wired. No more Wi-Fi.

In Los Angeles and other cities in the United States, water and other energy utility companies had attempted to impose 'smart' wireless meters on customers unilaterally, including the use of police in certain cases, and households had reported a string of adverse physical reactions in previously healthy adults, children and even pets. The companies backed down, switching to a 'voluntary' meter installation policy and faced a string of multi-million dollar class action lawsuits.

British utility companies were planning the installation of similar 'smart' meters around the country, without customer consultation and with the consent of government. ES-UK, Radiation Research Trust and MCS-AWARE had commissioned Dr Isaac Jamieson's 'Smart Meters – Smarter Practices' report on wireless health problems, which Brian Stein, Eileen O'Connor, Dr Erica Mallery-Blythe and others handed in to Number 10, Downing Street.

Within a short time, questions were tabled in the House of Commons and a government minister would announce that smart meters would not be made compulsory in Britain. The *Daily Telegraph* described this as 'a wise move.'

Less than four years earlier, in his meeting with Justice Minister Kenneth Clark, Brian Stein had been called 'a troublemaker and a conspiracy theorist' and shown the door. This time, was the message being taken more seriously?

3 Into the Electrostorm

'We are an electrochemical soup at the cellular and organ level. Think of ECG (electrocardiogram), EEG (electroencephalogram), and EMG (electromyogram). We evolved in a complex EMF environment with an interplay of natural terrestrial and extra-terrestrial EMF sources from solar activity, cosmic rays, and geomagnetic activity. I believe that our evolutionary balance, developed over the millennia, has been severely disturbed and disrupted by man-made EMFs.'

'The very good news is that there are reasonable ways to eliminate or reduce this hazard if society chooses to do so, in ways that can make modern life far safer without requiring us to live in the dark.'

– Dr Samuel Milham *'Dirty Electricity'*

By 2012, there were 1.9 billion mobile phone users and 5 million microwave masts worldwide. Wi-Fi was the technological miracle that had revolutionised social interaction, joined up businesses and emancipated young and old, great and small, rich and poor, regardless of race, creed or colour. What was not to like?

'Mobile Radiation ups cancer risk'

'The 450,000 mobile towers in India are turning the country into an open microwave,' warned Professor Girish Kumar, a faculty member of the Electrical Engineering Department at IIT in Mumbai.

Professor Kumar was speaking at a seminar on mobile phone and tower radiation attended by researchers, industry figures and members of the Department of Technology, Science and the Environment. Citing a case study where six residents of a Mumbai high-rise were affected by cancer, he said that mobile phone companies were compromising on public safety in installing higher intensity masts to cut costs: 'Those living in a 50-300 metre radius face a high risk much worse than smoking as you cannot see or smell radiation,' he said, 'you cannot have coincidence everywhere.'

Kumar believed that the Specific Absorption Rate (SAR) in India had been set at a far higher level than was safe in order to benefit the telecom operators who contributed 30% of the nation's GDP. Setting the rate at a lower and safer level would mean installing more masts at a higher cost. To Kumar, this was a price worth paying:

'Biological effects include drying of fluids around the eyes, the brain, heart and abdomen... sleep disruption, headaches, lack of concentration and memory loss... prolonged exposure to mobile radiation increases the chances of cancer by 200-400% over eight to ten years... It can also lead to miscarriages.'

All of this was at odds with the 'no short-term effects' posture in the UK of the likes of Professor Lawrie Challis.

Industry response to Kumar's assertions at the seminar was limited, with the head of one Indian telecom company saying that the risks were insignificant, or non-existent: adding that in any case there had to be a 'trade-off' between the benefits and ill-effects of mobiles.

A month later, however, on 8 and 9 February, 2012, at a workshop on 'Testing and Compliance for EMF in the Mobile Industry' at the 'Ensuring Public Health and Safety in the Mobile Industry' conference in New Delhi, Professor Kumar's awkward questions provoked the might of ICNIRP and the mobile industry's public relations machine.

When ICNIRP Chairman Dr Paolo Vecchia declared that ICNIRP guidelines for radiation density of 9.2 W/m squared were valid for 'one day, one year and even one hundred years of exposure', Professor Kumar asked him: 'Shall we expose you to 9.2 W/m squared for one year?'

The response from Dr Vecchia was silence, and the session chair intervened to say that Professor Kumar 'did not mean it.' Professor Kumar replied that he did mean it, and cited numerous reports and reports on reports which in his opinion backed up his findings, including one entitled *'The Impact of Communication Towers on Wildlife'* submitted by ten eminent Indian scientists to the Ministry of the Environment, which referred to 919 papers, out of which 563 concluded there was an impact, 130 decided there was none and the remainder were inconclusive.

The response of the foreign delegates, according to Professor Kumar, was that the Indian scientists were 'biased' and that they 'referred more papers which showed there is impact.'

Next up was Dr C.K Chou, Chairman of the IEEE and scourge of Professor Om P. Gandhi and others who had once toed the mobile industry line, but now refuted IEEE and ICNIRP safety levels. During the course of the day and the following day, Dr Chou reiterated the IEEE and ICNIRP safety levels for masts and cell phones, and asked why India wanted them tightened: why not have one 'harmonised' standard 'like one sun in the sky'?

Professor Kumar's reaction suggested not only a difference of scientific opinion, but an unwillingness to be trampled over by American cultural homogenisation: *'Why not adopt the safest radiation level as one global standard, rather than a standard which is valid only for the short term?'*

Furthermore: *'When we talk about one sun, the same sun is not present in the USA when it is present in India. Even when the same sun is present in India, its effect across the length and breadth of the country is not the same.'*

His subsequent questions to Dr Chou were *'simply brushed aside... I am not sure whether it was arrogance and/or ignorance.'*

As the conference drew to a close, Professor Kumar began to detect a pattern in the presentations: the industry was repeating itself time and again. He had been invited to participate in the final panel discussion: suddenly this was cancelled 'due to paucity of time.'

The theme of the conference was 'Ensuring Public Heath and Safety in the Mobile Industry'. So where were the public? Professor Kumar identified five possible members of the public out of 150 people in the audience. And where, he asked himself, were the likes of Professor Olle Johansson, Leif Salford and Allan Frey?

'It became obvious that the foreign delegates had a simple agenda: if India adopts a better radiation norm, then several other countries will also start demanding a better radiation norm. So, let India maintain ICNIRP guidelines and let people be exposed to high radiation 24/7. Do these foreign delegates… really care about the health of the Indian people? I have never seen any meeting conducted and concluded like this before.'

'The time has come, when people have to wake up and realise associated health hazards from cell phone and cell tower radiations. The sooner they realise, the better it will be: otherwise, the high radiation from cell towers will affect millions of people, birds, animals, the fruit yield of trees, plants and the environment.'

He also learned that the conference had been sponsored by Vodafone.

Brian Stein's Diary, 2012

On 16 January, after a combination of 'flu and ES symptoms I had a day off ill, the first in 16 years. Which makes me feel rather defeated because being ES while being told it's psychosomatic and scaremongering used by malingerers, you become very sensitive to that and try not to have time off. So in my 16 years and 10 years of being ES this is the first time.

*

In January 2012, in Benjarafe, Spain, after two years of local complaint and industry appeal, an unlicensed Vodafone mast was to be taken down in a 'cancer cluster' village.

Electromagnetic Health reported on a new study by Adamantia Fragapopolou and others showing that radiation from mobile and cordless phones below ICNIRP heating safety levels caused changes in the proteins that influence learning and memory in rats' brains:

'We have demonstrated that 143 proteins are altered after electromagnetic radiation, including proteins that have been correlated so far with Alzheimer's glioblastoma, stress and metabolism. In its perspective, this study is anticipated to throw light in the understanding of such health effects like headaches, dizziness, sleep disorders, memory disorders, brain tumours, all of them related, to the function of the altered brain proteins.'

Professor Margaritis added: *'The message taken out of this work is that people should be very cautious when using mobile phones next to their body (especially next to their brain), whereas the wireless DECT should be located as far away as possible from places that people use to spend many hours a day, not to mention children of all ages.'*

Professor Yury Grigoriev reported on a four-year study comparing children aged 7-12 using mobiles with others that showed *'an increase in phonemic perception disorders, abatement of efficiency, reduced indicators for the arbitrary and semantic memory and increased fatigue.'*

Profesor Olle Johansson of the Karolinska Institute in Stockholm wrote to the Environment Committee in Dublin: *'The present risk assessment of EMFs, such as mobile phone radiation, is scientifically untenable. It is therefore high time to abandon the pseudo-scientific risk assessment methodology that industry-sponsored top experts have designed to benefit industry interests at the expense of public health.'*

Dr Andrew Tresidder was a General Practitioner in Somerset, England. Dr Tresidder wrote an open letter to colleagues and other GPs:

'Electrosensitivity is an invisible, but very real problem for many people... It is caused by the interaction of artificial electromagnetic fields with biological systems, both from field effects from cables and appliances, and from transmission effects from transmitting technology. Mechanisms are thought to include calcium efflux from cells, interference with the blood-brain barrier, general sympathetic upregulation, and interference with free radical pair recombination amongst others.'

'A number of my patients have symptoms and illnesses which have been caused by exposure to electromagnetic fields, and which have been relieved by avoidance of the same fields.'

In South Korea, at the Department of Life Science and Institute for Natural Sciences, Hanyang University, Seoul, Gye and Park's paper was accepted on 'Effect of electromagnetic field exposure on the reproductive system'.

'Humans in modern society are exposed to an ever-increasing number of electromagnetic fields (EMFs) generated from the production and supply of electricity, television (TV) sets, personal computer (PC), radio communication, and mobile communication. Since the 1960s, when the biological hazard of EMF was studied in the Soviet Union, the safety of humans exposed to EMFs both at home and during occupational activities has become an important issue in public health. The biological effects of EMFs are currently under debate and still a controversial issue. In the present review, the effects of EMFs on reproductive function are summarized according to the types of EMFs and duration of exposure at the cellular and organism levels...'

'Through in vitro and in vivo studies, MF exposure was found to alter the reproductive endocrine hormones, gonadal function, embryonic development, pregnancy, and fetal development... These effects were different according to the frequency, duration of exposure, and strength of EMFs. Humans in modern society cannot avoid various kinds of EMFs during household and occupational activities, but should be aware of the biological hazard of EMFs. The effort to avoid EMF exposure and techniques *to protect or relieve EMF radiation are required to preserve our reproductive potential.'*

Brian Stein's Diary, 8 March 2012

Met up with two solicitors to discuss electrosensitivity and possibility of a legal case. They're frightened to death of the mobile phone industry! Not in the UK!

Early April, 2012: Retired from 17 years in Samworth Brothers. They gave me a very good send off and we'll see whether or not not working helps or hinders my ES.

Brian Stein had already put his weight behind the ES-UK cause. He became Chairman of the Radiation Research Trust and was a trustee of ES-UK, with around 1,000 members, many of whom were isolated by and from wireless communications and received the ES-UK newsletter and other information in hard copy form.

In April, 2012, Michael Repacholi, former head of the World Health Organisation EMF project and Chairman Emeritus of ICNIRP, continued to attack his former WHO boss Gro Harlem Brundtland for speaking out about her electrosensitivity and her warnings about mobile phones.

In an interview with Norwegian journalist Thomas Ergo, Repacholi described her disclosure as 'unfortunate' and suggested she had contributed 'massively' to people's fears of wireless radiation from mobile phones – which indeed had been Dr Brundtland's stated intention.

Following publication of the interview in *Aftenbladet*, a daily newspaper, two senior Norwegian legislators were quoted as defending Dr Brundtland against Repacholi's assertion that electrosensitivity was a 'psychosocial' rather than a medical condition: 'I believe people who say they are allergic to mobile phone radiation' said a member of the Parliament's heath committee.

If Repacholi's pursuit of Dr Brundtland seemed dogged to the point of pathological, Dr Brundtland was not about to yield under his pressure. A week later, addressing the opening of the new School of Public Health and Health Systems at the University of Waterloo in Canada, her mobile phone rang during her presentation. Dr Brundtland removed it from her purse, told the audience the call was from Oslo and that she would answer it later. She then held up the phone and said that it was a Blackberry, which had been invented at Waterloo, the city where they were gathered, before continuing her address.

Afterwards, questions were invited from the audience. Dr Magda Havas worked at Trent University with people who believed they were suffering from electrohypersensitivity. She asked Dr Brundtland what advice she had for the University of Waterloo and the rest of Canada:

'I assume you know I am electrically sensitive,' Dr Brundtland replied, 'I never place a mobile phone next to my head because in one second I would develop a bad headache. I use the phone in speaker mode.'

Dr Brundtland went on to describe how she had become electrically sensitive after the domestic incident with a microwave oven: 'I have been heavily criticised as scaring people from using cell phones because I have told the truth about my illness,' she went on. 'This is important. We are exposed to different technologies of a new nature. I am frustrated that I was unable to sound the alarm fully. A single sentence in an instruction book – where you do not explain (in greater depth) the danger of radio frequency – is not good public health and consumer policy.'

'I became electrically sensitive and have been criticised because I can scare the public. We know they are not inert and there are potential consequences. People who have electrical sensitivity show that we do take some risk. Until we know more, we cannot say this is no problem.'

'Let your children have a mobile phone all day?' she concluded, 'No!'

Meanwhile, a Japanese study of 18,000 teenage children indicated links between their after lights-out mobile phone usage, poor sleep quality and even suicidal thoughts.

No Refuge

Michael Nield's family had already moved from Herefordshire 150 miles east to the remote Cambridgeshire village of Wardy Hill, where they hoped he and his mother would be less affected by the electromagnetic fields they believed were making Michael's life in particular a misery. Mobile phones, he said, gave him 'a constant zapping' in his head.

An Oxford graduate and a talented violinist, he slept with a microfibre tent over his bed and wore a micro-mesh body suit when he went out, both of which seemed to ameliorate the effects of microwaves on his body.

'He tried everything to get better,' his mother said, 'he sought help, he ate a specific diet and he tried so hard.' This was not enough: on 3 June, 2012, Michael's father Clive found his son's car parked on a grass track near the family home. Michael was inside: he had killed himself with a cocktail of drugs and alcohol.

'Unless people have electrosensitivity they just don't realise what sort of effects it has,' his mother said at the inquest, 'We saw it (moving here) as a positive step, but looking back it was his last-ditch attempt to be normal and put his illness aside. But that was obviously something he couldn't do.'

Had they been able to communicate, Michael Nield and Phil Inkley might at least have had some words of support. The irony was that the default media of everyday communications – wireless masts and mobile phones – were the very triggers of their isolation and distress.

Inkley had been a sound technician, and in his own words an enthusiastic 'techie' always on hand to fix friends' and family's computers. However, after days surrounded by Wi-Fi he began to experience pressure on his temples and pains in his chest. The symptoms repeated when he tuned in his father's hands-free mobile phone kit.

'I looked online at some reports on EHS from independent scientists,' he recalled, 'I didn't like what I was reading, so I tried to leave it alone.'

As his symptoms worsened, Phil Inkley 'wanted to believe I was going mad. It would have been easier. But I knew I wasn't. I hoped for a while that gas boiler was leaking carbon monoxide and giving me headaches. But it wasn't.'

By this time he was experiencing nosebleeds, dizziness and blackouts. His GP told him that there was no compelling evidence that these symptoms could be caused by electromagnetic fields: 'I was getting really scared about what was happening to me, but I thought, 'This is England, I'll just get in touch with the authorities and explain, and they'll sort it out.'

Inkley made several calls to the UK Health Protection Agency, each time leaving a voicemail: each time, answer came there none. Eventually, he received a voicemail: don't call us again.

Desperate to reduce his symptoms, he moved to a caravan in a remote part of Hampshire. On bad days he withdrew still further to an abandoned children's den in the woods and cooked over an open fire. His symptoms persisted and with them his sense of fear and personal isolation:

'I've been through hellishly desperate times with this,' he told a reporter, 'People don't believe that EMFs are the cause of EHS, and it gets you in such a state. You're battling for your existence, and people think it's all in your head.'

In one sense, people were right: it *was* in his head, just as it had been in the heads of Michael Nield and many others. Beyond the Hampshire woods, the proposition that the sources, however, lay *outside* his head was gaining currency.

*

In Sweden, Michael Carlberg and Lennart Hardell of the Department of Oncology, University Hospital Orebro, supported by funding from Cancer-och Allergifunden, Cancerhjalpen and Orebro University Hospital Cancer Fund, published their report: *'On the association between glioma, wireless phones, heredity and non-ionising radiation'.*

The report reiterated the methodological flaws in the Danish study recently republished in the BMJ, and concluded: *'Certainly results from the Hardell-group as well as from the Interphone group show an increased risk for glioma associated with long term mobile 'phone use. Also use of cordless phones increases the risk when properly assessed and analysed. The risk is highest for ipsilateral exposure to the brain of RF-EMF emissions. Adolescents seem to be at higher risk than adults. IARC concluded that RF-MF emissions overall, eg occupational and from wireless phones, are 'possibly carcinogenic to humans, Group 2B.'*

In August, 2012, Professor Yury Grigoriev, Deputy Chairman of the Russian National Committee on Non-Ionising Radiation Protection and Director of the Centre for Electromagnetic Safety, issued a statement: *'Man conquered the Black Plague, but he has created new problems – EMF Pollution.'*

Grigoriev was one of Russia's most distinguished scientists and an authority on the biological effects of non-ionising and ionising radiation, a field in which he had worked since 1949. He had been closely associated with the Soviet Space Programme and was a leading member of the Government Commission on the 1986 Chernobyl accident. He had published fifteen books, over three hundred papers in referred journals and supervised over seventy successful doctoral dissertations. He had also attended the 2008 Radiation Research Trust Conference in London:

'The brain is a critical organ,' Grigoriev said, 'Vital brain structures are under EMF exposure daily when using a mobile phone. The brain is made up of permanent complex biophysical processes and vital functions. We need to take care with mobile phones and use distance and reduce time,' adding that children should limit their mobile phone use and adults should use hands-free.

Russian researchers stood by their findings that cognitive function in humans and animals was disturbed by prolonged exposure to microwave radiation, and rejected as inadequate both the current ICNIRP safety thresholds and the 'thermal-only' view of the biological hazards from masts and mobiles. The Russian government issued health warnings to pregnant women and children under eighteen, cautioning also of the effects on future generations.

Grigoriev's statements, given his personal authority and coupled with the imminent release of the Russian research in English, were greeted with elation in ES research circles in London and Stockholm. The UK Radiation Research Trust's Eileen O'Connor and her colleague Sissel Halmoy, Chairman of the International EMF Alliance and Secretary-General of Citizens Radiation Protection in Norway, went to Russia to visit him.

'The Russian report is a gift to the world,' said O'Connor, 'Russian scientists are advanced in their knowledge of RF/EMF radiation and have extended the hand of friendship and are willing to share their expertise and knowledge. I hope decision-makers from the western world accept this great honour and work together.'

Eileen O'Connor lived in Wishaw, Lancashire, where she had been diagnosed in 2001 with breast cancer when she was 37 years old:

'I'd go along to consultations and there were all these relatively young women there like me, and I thought, what's going on?'

O'Connor discovered that six women had been diagnosed within eighteen months, all of whom lived within 500 metres of a T-Mobile microwave mast. In addition to her own symptoms, her hitherto healthy son had begun to develop nosebleeds: 'Then they applied to put up more masts, and I thought, hang on a minute… so we hit the phones.'

What happened thereafter was reminiscent of the film *Calendar Girls* without the nudity. O'Connor and her friends turned themselves from cancer 'victims' into a media-savvy force for change: 'And in 2005, the mast came down. The industry hated it – we had out-publicised them in every medium.'

The T-Mobile mast was delivered to a local scrapyard, where it was broken up. Never ones to miss ramming home a point, O'Connor and her colleagues put out a press release: *'Piece of Mast, Peace of Mind.'*

With Alasdair Phillips of Powerwatch, she attended a mobile phone industry conference where ICNIRP's Mike Repacholi was centre stage.

'He was saying 'It's safe' and everyone was agreeing with him. So I was in the front row and Alasdair was in the back row, and we started asking the awkward questions.'

'I shall never forget the look Repacholi gave me – it was a look of pure hatred - and he continued to focus it on me throughout the session.'

In 2008, she had helped Brian Stein organise the inaugural Radiation Research Trust conference in London, again including Mike Repacholi.

'His line was still, 'it's safe'. When you really get to know him, I think he realises there's a problem.'

The 2012 meeting in Russia between Eileen O'Connor, Sissel Halmoy and Professor Yury Grigoriev was a meeting of minds in more than one sense. Sissel Halmoy was a rocket scientist, who had worked on missile guidance systems. She had been electrically sensitive for twenty-seven years.

'Electrosensitivity breaks up happy families,' she observed, having 'swept' her London hotel with an acoustimeter in order to find a room with the lowest intensity electromagnetic field.

Of the mobile phone industry, she said: 'There is a 'bad experts' group of scientists. We are not allowed to be in it – they only choose their own friends.'

'This is a criminal story – it's not about science. There's a war going on.'

In Britain, Iain Duncan-Smith MP agreed to present the English translation of Professor Grigoriev's findings to the United Kingdom's Chief Medical Officer, Professor Dame Sally Davies.

This was more than a report on smart meters handed in by a few campaigners to 10 Downing Street. Would the British Government, for so long led by America in matters mobile as in so many other matters, and Professor Dame Sally Davies, listen to Professor Grigoriev as well as, or even instead of, ICNIRP and the UK Health Protection Agency?

Brian Stein's Diary, 4 September 2012

Final endoscopy and all clear.

This was good news – and vindication of the lengths to which he had gone to minimise his exposure to EMFs.

Stein was one of the business leaders who chaired and mentored the Common Purpose forums for young professionals held in central London. Today's theme was 'Courage and Caution'. He decided to adjust the agenda.

'I'm not going to talk about leadership, or caution,' he told them, 'I'm going to talk about electrosensitivity.'

'In September 2000 I started to have weird sensations while I was on my mobile. I went to see my GP. When you're a Chief Executive dealing with Tesco and Sainsburys, the whole of your credibility is about being a sane human being - you keep quiet.'

A ripple of unease went around the room – this was a volunteer audience of youngsters keen to learn the secrets of success from a business leader. But no-one was about to get up and leave.

Stein told them about Professor Fothergill. He told them about how he 'came out' in the *Daily Telegraph* 'and exposed myself as a nutcase'. He told them about Chief Inspector Strong. His Liverpudlian vowels and self-deprecating delivery were beginning to reach the audience.

'If somebody like myself is not prepared to stand up and speak out,' he said, 'who will?'

He quoted from the health warnings buried in the small print in Blackberry manual – at which point some of the audience glanced at their mobile phones strewn around the table.

The first question came: 'So are you arguing against mobile phones?'

'No, but it might come across as that.'

Stein cited the work of Dr Lennart Hardell and the health warnings in the Swiss government handbook. He cited the UK Health Protection Agency's record on cigarettes and asbestos; and international progress in recognising the issue of ES and EMFs as opposed to lack of recognition in the UK and United States.

The audience were cautious, but they were thinking.

'I'm a physicist,' said one, 'I'm not surprised at your story. But there are a lot of doubters out there. How are you going to take this forward?'

'I chair the RRT and am a trustee of ES-UK. I try to disseminate the human side and the science. And the problem is that it requires an awful lot of both. We're speaking to the French, the Swedes, the Americans... the Americans are becoming a little bit more interested.'

'The mood around the world is beginning to change – in India for example. Sadly not in the UK.'

Stein produced a microwave detector and the room started as it rose in volume: 'Sometimes I do this and ask someone to make a mobile phone call – then people really jump.'

He was having a greater effect on the room: 'Do I see changes? Yes - but it's very, very slow. The last time I did a talk, in Nottingham, it had gone from around zero to around 20% of people saying, 'Yes, I think I have a problem – my phone affects me.'

'The truth is that when you are trying to do something as dramatic as this, it is going to be slow. The alternative is to do nothing, or go mad.'

'We are going to have to embarrass the UK Health Protection Agency.'

Another question: 'Why should people believe you?'

'All I would say is this – the majority of the research by far that is not sponsored by the mobile phone industry shows that it is not safe.'

'Where do you draw the courage from?'

'It was simply worthwhile to be proven right… however much people ridicule you behind your back.'

'Our cells have never experienced this volume of information carried on the wavelengths before.'

'Before you can get anywhere you have to recognise that there's a problem – once you recognise that, man is very ingenious and will find a way around these things.'

The session ended after two hours. In a café afterwards, Brian Stein answered more questions and told the story of the successful businesswoman whose BMW 7 Series was causing her trouble because she was electrically sensitive. He had given her some advice about what car to buy.

'Thanks, 'she said. 'Oh by the way, don't call me, I'll call you.'

'Okay, why's that?'

'It's my husband. He won't allow me to be ES.'

*

In September, 2012, in Greece, Dr Dimitris Panagopoulos of the University of Athens released research suggesting that the effects of microwave exposure to cells were more threatening than previously supposed, and greater than 'natural' threats. This was the latest in the growing number of independent studies suggesting that exposure to microwave radiation on the current scale could result in damage to DNA in future generations, and ultimately even a failure to reproduce: a view shared by scientists such as Professor Olle Johansson.

Israel removed electric cars from its police force. Research into EMFs was under way in India and China. In Germany, an electric clock user manual included warnings for ES people. In Italy, the Vatican was in conflict with villagers who objected to the emissions from one of its wireless masts.

An Italian court upheld the 2009 Innocenzo Marcolini case verdict linking mobile phone use to his brain tumour. The judge cited Professor Lennart Hardell's research as the gold standard science – a phrase privately used of Hardell by US scientists - in pronouncing judgement, and the fact that Hardell was not funded by the mobile phone industry.

Why else had Innocenzo Marcolini succeeded where others like David Reynard in the United States had so far failed? Unlike in America and the UK, among other countries, the Italian government had tightened mobile phone safety thresholds to the point where successful litigation was possible. This local legal precedent subverted the 'one size fits all' assertion of C.K Chou, Mike Repacholi and ICNIRP and was only the first of its kind.

In India, new regulations would be rolled out regarding cell phones. The Vodafone conference in New Delhi attended by Professor Kumar, funded and heavily populated by the mobile industry, had, it seemed, failed to carry the day.

Brian Stein's Diary, 10 December 2012

I showed the Italian Supreme Court (Marcolini) ruling to a legal person in the UK. They were shocked – they couldn't believe that it could happen and that people would not know about it in the

UK. The Italian Court did not accept the ICNIRP evidence – they thought it was tainted and they believed Lennart Hardell's work.

2013, Belgium: Not in My Boardroom

Didier Bellens caused some surprise when he ordered Wi-Fi to be banned from his 27th floor management offices, and asked contacts to call him on his landline rather than his mobile. Bellens was President of Belgacom, Belgium's largest mobile phone company.

At an event organised by Child Focus and Microsoft, he also took the opportunity to tell children at the Centre of Woluwe-Saint-Pierre School about the dangers of GSM (Global System for Mobile Communications): 'During the day, it is better to use a headset because the GSM, it heats,' he told them, 'The waves are dangerous. At night, it is better to shut it off. If you use your phone as an alarm clock, you should also turn it off.'

Bellens was almost certainly aware that proposed legislation was imminent in Belgium banning the sale of mobile phones to children under seven years of age, and advertising controlled to those under fourteen. As head of Belgacom, he could thus be seen to acting 'responsibly' in the interests of himself, his company and the community. Nevertheless, this did not deter a Belgacom spokesperson.

'Didier Bellens is only indicating the precautionary principles recommended by the World Health Organisation. Remember that nothing has ever been proven about the dangers of GSM…'

Shortly afterwards, on 28 February, 2013, the Belgian Public Health Minister Laurent Onkelinx announced the proposed measures in question, citing the high incidence of mobile phone use – two out of every three children under ten years old - and the dangers of microwave radiation on the child's developing brain. Belgian parents presumably in many cases reacted with approval at the announcement - and with trepidation at how their offspring would react in turn.

*

The latest Bioinitiative Working Group report assembled research data from over 1,600 studies and concluded that risks to health from electromagnetic fields and wireless technologies had substantially increased since 2007. Cell phone users, parents-to-be, young children and pregnant women were particularly at risk.

Professor Lennart Hardell put it bluntly: 'Epidemiological evidence shows that radiofrequency should be classified as a human carcinogen. The FCC/IEEE and ICNIRP public safety limits and reference levels are not adequate to protect public health.'

Hardell particularly pointed to the pattern of increased risk of glioma, or malignant brain tumour, and acoustic neuroma, with the use of mobile and cordless phones. Also:

'A dozen new studies link cell phone radiation to sperm damage. Even a cell phone in the pocket or on a belt may harm sperm DNA, result in misshapen sperm, and impair fertility in men. Laptop computers with wireless internet connections can damage DNA in sperm.'

The consequences included altered brain development in the fetus and increased incidences of autism. As David O. Carpenter MD, co-editor of the report put it: *'There is now much more evidence to health affecting billions of people worldwide. The* status quo *is not acceptable in the light of the evidence of harm.'*

The Bioinitiative Report covered the effects of electromagnetic fields from power lines, electrical wiring, domestic appliances and handheld devices; also cell phones and cordless phones, cell phone masts and towers, 'smart meters', Wi-Fi, wireless laptops, wireless routers and baby monitors. The health hazards listed included damage to DNA and genes, loss of memory, reduced cognitive function, attention deficit behaviour, sleep disruption, cancer and Alzheimer's disease.

In China, they were reaching their own conclusions.

Hong Kong, 3 February, 2013

'Mobile phone antennae removed from university over cancer fears'

'Campus dwellers assured radiation exposure 'extremely low', but not all are convinced'

The students and staff of the University of Science and Technology might have been expected to welcome the miracle of microwave mobile technology, and indeed they did so in terms of their personal habits. However the appearance of an estimated 87 wireless microwave masts on the roofs of residential and student blocks in return for a reputed payment to the university from mobile phone companies caused consternation among residents versed in the scientific literature reporting links between microwave masts and cancer clusters:

'The WHO study refers to regular mobile phone use, not 24/7 exposure to mobile phone antennae,' said one member of staff, 'We are exposed to EMR day and night in our homes, offices, classrooms and student halls.'

Another member of staff challenged the claim that only one in three masts was in use: 'How does it make sense to keep erecting more masts if they will not be used?'

Faculty members called for the university to reveal the precise sum paid by the mobile phone companies: a university spokesperson declined to mention figures, but said that the money 'went to a university scholarship fund'.

As workmen began dismantling some of the masts, some members of the university with young children were not reassured: 'If these antennae are perfectly safe, why are they taking some of them down all of a sudden?' said one, speaking on condition of anonymity.

'Routine maintenance and cabling improvement works are carried out on an ongoing basis,' came the university's reply, 'If any antennae are found to be defective during this process, they may be removed and replaced.'

Brussels, 20 February, 2013

The UK Radiation Research Trust's Eileen O'Connor was among those attending the European Commission Unit D3's 'Workshop on Risk Communication – Electromagnetic Fields and Human Health' convened by Director-General Sanco. The Director-General was at pains to remind delegates that communication, and not management of risk, was the agenda: the Commission was 'not in a position' to deal with the Precautionary Principle established by Sir William Stewart, first ignored, then ridiculed and attacked by the industry, and now becoming enshrined in public health policy around the world.

Eileen O'Connor did not see his point: 'How,' she asked, does the Commission intend to provide risk communication without discussing the risks?'

O'Connor reiterated the growing public concern about health risks from exposure to electromagnetic fields: from base stations, Wi-Fi, smart meters and mobile phones. The Commission, she said, needed to review the latest evidence and take the latest findings into account. It was not ethical to expose the public to electromagnetic fields labelled as '2B possible human carcinogen' without informing them of the risks.

She cited Section 4.3.4 of The Precautionary principle under Article 174 EU Treaty (previously Article 130 before the Treaty renumbered). Article 174(2) stated: *'Community policy on the environment shall aim at a high level of protection taking into account the diversity of situations in the various regions of the Community. It shall be based on the precautionary principle and on the principles that preventive action should be taken.'*

'Environmental damage should as a priority be rectified at source and that the polluter should pay.'

The EU, 'Connor declared, was 'totally ignoring and misusing the Precautionary Principle and this approach is forcing the public to take action into their own hands via the courts and through spreading information and research via action groups.

Lack of action and consideration from authorities and policy makers is creating the need for a global movement amongst activists. There are now approximately 85 organisations listed under the umbrella for the International EMF Alliance and the list is growing.'

She cited the Marcolini judgement in Italy, and the judgement of a Spanish Labour Court which ruled on the 'permanent incapacitation' of a college professor who suffered from chronic fatigue and environmental and electromagnetic hypersensitivity. Both judgements rejected industry-funded studies that claimed mobile phones and radio frequency radiation were safer than independently-funded studies such as those by Professor Lennart Hardell reported them to be.

Policy makers, she added, were 'clearly failing to catch up with the science, the courts and public opinion.' Measures needed to be taken as a matter of urgency to alert the public to the latest information.

The continued lack of action or implementation of the precautionary approach to RF from the EU Commission and other authorities was also leading to serious frustration on the part of some politicians, many doctors and independent scientists, many of the latter of whom were now refusing to attend meetings at the EU Commission due to the lack of attention shown towards their advice or opinions.

Prominent among them was Professor Denis Henshaw of Bristol University:

'The mis-match between our extensive scientific knowledge of the adverse health effects of exposures to EMFs of all forms, and the unwillingness of Governments including the EU even to listen to the scientific advice from those most knowledgeable in the field, well illustrates the unwillingness of many to attend the EMF workshop on risk communication.'

The business risks for investors in companies listed on the New York Stock Exchange were also discussed in the annual report of the Securities Exchange Act of 1934 for the fiscal year ending December 21, 2011.

The report included the following statement from VERIZON, the US subsidiary of mobile giant Vodafone:

'Our wireless business also faces personal injury and consumer class action lawsuits relating to alleged health effects of wireless phones or radio frequency transmitters, and class action lawsuits that challenge marketing practices and disclosures relating to alleged adverse health effects of handheld wireless phones. We may incur significant expenses in defending these lawsuits. In addition, we may be required to pay significant awards or settlements.'

The following year, in 2014, Vodafone would complete the disposal of its holding in Verizon, trumpeting the return of a record dividend to its shareholders. Was this the real agenda behind the sale?

Meanwhile, back at Microsoft, February's UK Hotmail 'Welcome' page featured a 'happy and healthy' young mother and daughter on the bed, a wireless laptop planted in the daughter's lap, pulsing microwaves into the little girl's pre-pubescent reproductive organs.

*

On 28 February, 2013, an Australian court ruled that Comcare, the government agency charged with enforcing worker safety laws, should pay compensation to Dr David McDonald for damage to his health during his employment by the Commonwealth Scientific and Industrial Research Organisation caused by exposure to electromagnetic fields. This was the first legal acknowledgement of electrohypersensitivity in Australia.

The Judge, Deputy President JW Constance, ruled that he was 'satisfied on the balance of probabilities that Dr McDonald has suffered either an aggravation of his sensitivity to EMF, or an aggravation of his symptoms by reason of his honest belief that he suffers from the condition of EMF sensitivity.'

'I am satisfied,' the judge went on, 'that the ailment from which Dr McDonald suffers is not itself a perception. In this case the perceptions, if any, of Dr McDonald are that the disorder (and therefore the ailment) from which he suffers is caused by exposure to EMF and that the aggravation of the disorder was caused by his exposure to EMF during the trials carried out by his employer.'

In Israel, a world leader in IT with a population among the heaviest cell phone users in the world, on 3 March, 2013, the local Orange network operator Partner agreed to pay 400,000 shekels (approximately US $100,000) to a lawyer who sued the company on the grounds that he had developed a rare and aggressive lymphoma near his left ear after using two cell phones he had bought from the company. The lawyer had converted the 'secure room' – the bomb shelter featured in most new Israeli homes – in his house to an office from where he conducted business including a great many mobile phone calls. The electromagnetic radiation from mobile phones was higher than usual in places such as these with low reception, and mobiles marketed in Israel carried explicit warnings including the avoidance of use in such places.

Unlike the Marcolini case in Italy and Dr McDonald in Australia, the Israeli laywer's suit for damages was rejected by the court. Partner maintained that it was 'very meticulous about adhering to the guidelines of the World Health Organisation, the Health Ministry, the Communications Ministry and all relevant bodies', and was making the one-off settlement 'as a humanitarian gesture'. Nevertheless, it was suggested by many that a precedent had been created for further lawsuits to be brought by mobile phone users who believed they had developed cancers as a result of exposure to EMFs.

*

The American corporation had developed the mobile phone: the American consumer was leading the way.

'FOR IMMEDIATE RELEASE: MARCH 7, 2013:'

'LA Teacher's Union Passes Resolution to Ensure Safety from Hazardous Electromagnetic Fields (EMF) in Schools including EMF Emissions from Wireless Technology'

'United Teachers Los Angeles (UTLA), representing over 40,000 teachers and other workers in LAUSD, passed the following motion by a sweeping majority last night at 9 PM (Motion for the new UTLA Resolution transcribed from attendee, Shane Gregory's transcripts):'

'**Health and Human Services Committee 3-6-13 #1:** Moved by Kevin Mottus, seconded by John Cabrera.'

"I move that UTLA will abide by current **National NEA Policy for Environmentally Safe Schools** which states that all employees and stakeholders should be informed when there are changes in their exposure to environmental hazards including electromagnetic radiation and that all stakeholders and the public should be notified of any actual and potential hazards. UTLA will advocate for technological solutions that maintain technology upgrades while not increasing employees exposure to electromagnetic radiation."

'Rationale: The NEA National Policy Resolution C-18 Environmentally Safe Schools states as follows:'

"C-18 Environmentally Safe Schools"

'The National Education Association believes that all educational facilities must have healthy indoor air quality, be smoke-free, and be safe from environmental and chemical hazards, <u>and from hazardous electromagnetic fields</u>...'

'<u>The Association further believes that school districts must inform all stakeholders when changes in their exposure to electromagnetic radiation occur</u>. Additional health hazards should not be created when facilities are altered or repaired.'

"The Association believes that school districts must post MSDS (Material Safety Data Sheets) and OSHA (Occupational Safety *and Health Administration) standards. <u>Students and/or their parents/guardians, education employees, and the public should be notified of actual and potential hazards</u>. All stakeholders should be involved in developing a plan for corrective action. The Association also believes in the development and enforcement of health and safety standards specifically for children. (1989, 2004)."*

"In May of 2011 based on the latest research, The World Health Organization classified electromagnetic fields as a Class 2B Carcinogen along with Lead and DDT. Current FCC guidelines for electromagnetic radiation explicitly do not cover children or pregnant women. According to NEA Policy our employees have the right to know about changes in their environment which may have adverse health effects."

'March 19, 2013'

'Los Angeles Unified School District'

'333 S Beaudry Ave #24'

'Los Angeles, CA 90017'

'The American Academy of Environmental Medicine comprises Medical Doctors, Osteopaths and PhD researchers focusing on the effects of environmental agents on human health. For forty years the Academy has trained Physicians to treat the most difficult, to heal patients who are often overlooked by our medical system because the cause of their illness is a chemical, solvent, or toxic metal, not a bacteria, virus or other traditionally understood cause.'

'In recent years our members and colleagues have reported an increase in patients whose symptoms are reversible by eliminating wireless radiating devices in their homes such as cell phones, cordless phones and wireless internet systems.'

'There is consistent emerging science that shows people, especially children, are affected by the increasing exposure to wireless radiation. In September 2010, the Journal of the American

Society for Reproductive Medicine – Fertility and Sterility reported that after only four hours of exposure to a standard laptop using Wi-Fi caused DNA damage to human sperm.'

'In October 2012, the AAEM issued a public warning about Wi-Fi in schools that stated:'

'Adverse health effects from wireless radio frequency fields, such as learning disabilities, altered immune responses, and headaches, clearly exist and are well documented in the scientific literature. Safer technology, such as hardwiring, is strongly recommended in schools.'

'In December 2012, the American Academy of Paediatrics representing 60,000 paediatricians -wrote to Congress requesting it update the safety levels of microwave radiation exposure especially for children and pregnant women:'

'The Wi-Fi systems in schools are typically hundreds of times more powerful than the home consumer systems you may be familiar with. They are also dozens of times more powerful than the café and restaurant systems you may have been exposed to. The Wi-Fi systems in schools are necessarily more powerful than any microwave communication systems in any other setting because they are required to run hundreds of computers simultaneously. They are also exposing children –the Los Angeles Unified School District most vulnerable to microwave radiation – to extended periods all day, for their entire childhood.'

'This is an unprecedented exposure with unknown outcome on the health and reproductive potential of a generation.'

'To install this system in Los Angeles risks a widespread public health question that the medical system is not yet prepared to answer.'

'In October 2013, the AAEM is organizing an international medical conference in Phoenix AZ to teach doctors how to identify patients whose symptoms can be reversed by eliminating exposure to Wi-Fi, cell phones and other forms of wireless radiation in the home.'

'It is unlikely that there are currently enough doctors in Los Angeles County familiar with the biological effects of microwave radiation to diagnose and treat the numbers of children who will potentially become symptomatic from exposure to your wireless system should you elect to install it. Statistics show that you can expect an immediate reaction in 3% of your students and time-delayed reactions in 30% of them. This will also include teachers.'

'The American Academy of Environmental Medicine suggests strongly that you do not add to the burden of public health by installing blanket wireless internet connections in Los Angeles schools. Hardwired internet connections are not only safer, they are stronger, and more secure.'

'Children who are required by law to attend school also require a higher level of protection than the general public. You may be directed by technology proponents that the science on the human health effects of Wi-Fi is not yet certain. This uncertainty is not a reason to subject a generation of children to such extreme exposure. Rather, it is the foundation upon which caution must be exercised to prevent a potential public health disaster.'

'While technicians and sales staff argue about the validity of the dangers posed by cell towers, cell phones, Wi-Fi and other forms of wireless radiation, it is the doctors who must deal with the fall out. Until we, as doctors, can determine why some of our patients become debilitatingly sick from Wi-Fi and other microwave communications, we implore you not to take such a known risk with the health of so many children who have entrusted you to keep them safe while at school.'

'Respectfully,'

'The Executive Committee of the American Academy of Environmental Medicine'

*

On 19 March, 2013, the Lower House of the French National Assembly voted an amendment of the law stipulating the use of 'hard wired' – ie Ethernet – connections over wireless connections in day care centres and pre-schools, the justification being the threat posed by microwave exposure from the latter to children's health.

This was the first time the 'precautionary principle' would be applied to French children. Supporters of the amendment noted that French mobile phone operators were still relying on the 2009 guidelines of the 'Agence Nationale de Securite Sanitaire' – the French equivalent of the UK Health Protection Agency – which, like its UK counterpart, was by default or design behind the curve of judicial thinking in Italy and Australia and independent scientific findings by the likes of Lennart Hardell.

Per Segerback in Sweden, the French air hostesses, Phil Inkley in England: these were individuals isolated and marginalised from the community. In Green Bank, West Virginia, in the United States, the challenge to the electromagnetic refugee was being met in the form of a community.

Refugees of the Modern World

'The "electrosensitive" are moving to a cell phone-free town. But is their disease real?'

'By Joseph Stromberg |Posted Friday, April 12, 2013, at 5:30 AM*

'You can turn your phone on in Green Bank, W.Va., but you won't get a trace of a signal. If you hit scan on your car's radio, it'll cycle through the dial endlessly, never pausing on a station. This remote mountainous town is inside the U.S. National Radio Quiet Zone, a 13,000–square-mile area where most types of electromagnetic radiation on the radio spectrum (which includes radio and TV broadcasts, Wi-Fi networks, cell signals, Bluetooth, and the signals used by virtually every other wireless device) are banned to minimize disturbance around the National Radio Astronomy Observatory, home to the world's largest steerable radio telescope.'

Diane and Bert Schou had lived healthily on their farm in Cedar Falls, Iowa. In 2002, US Cellular, a mobile operator, built a mast nearby. Diane took up the story: 'I was extremely tired, but I couldn't sleep at night,' she recalled, 'I got a rash, I had hair loss, my skin was wrinkled, and I just thought it was something I ate, or I was getting older.' Severe headaches followed, and Diane did some browsing online – whether via a hard-wired internet connection or courtesy of the mast, is not recorded. She learned about EHS and arranged a consultation with the world-famous Mayo Clinic: the doctors dismissed the possibility. She wrote to the FCC. Again, the response was brief: the mast was safe.

With her symptoms worsening, Diane Schou spent the next four years on repeated trips away from the farm, looking for places where they would abate. She drove more than 75,000 miles across the United States; she travelled through Scandinavia, where their son was studying. She found safe places – at first only US Cellular phones had triggered her symptoms. Then, proximity to almost any electrical device became a trigger: 'It would be like a sledgehammer on top of my head.'

In 2007, she heard about the Radio Quiet Zone.

She drove there and immediately felt better. She and Bert sold half their farm and bought a house in Green Bank, renovated it and installed wiring with thick insulation. Diane's symptoms abated. They put in a landline and a hard-wired computer connected to the internet. They couldn't find a refrigerator with low enough radiation emissions – all electrical devices emitted low-level radiation - so they installed an icebox which she filled by hand. Bert returned each summer to the farm.

The Schous' two-story brick house was four miles up a forest road: the nearest facility was Green Bank's post office. Even so, they kept a radiation meter in their living room. Diane's symptoms returned whenever she left the Radio Quiet Zone: 'I'll say, Oh, I have a headache, and then someone's cell phone will ring. This happens time and time again.'

'Life isn't perfect here,' she observed, 'there's no grocery store, no restaurants, no hospital. But here, at least, I'm healthy. I can do things. I'm not in bed with a headache all the time.'

Deborah Cooney was an economics alumna of Brown University, had been a vice president of People's Savings Bank of Massachussetts, and was now a singer, pianist and voice coach from Clairemont, San Diego, California. After a 'smart' electricity meter had been installed in her house and many others in 2010, her Frisbee champion boyfriend developed heart issues, she experienced dizziness, headaches, palpitations and sleeplessness, and even her cat started panting, pacing about and shaking her paws. Things got worse – she developed fatigue, numbness, circulation problems and heart pains – her boyfriend recovered, but her cat died. One night in October 2011, she moved out.

'I got so sick that I felt my life was in serious jeopardy, and if I didn't leave that minute, I didn't know if I'd survive,' she recalled.

Cooney left her boyfriend in the house and drove 2,600 miles across country to a friend in West Virginia who didn't have cell service, where she heard about the Radio Quiet Zone. She heard about Bert and Diane Schou, who took in other electromagnetic refugees. She moved into their home-built one-room cabin at the foot of their driveway. It had no running water or electricity, and she started feeling better. During the day, she started sharing an apartment nearby with another EHS person, where she could cook, bathe and occasionally use a computer.

There was no work locally: she travelled to gigs in Texas and Florida, sleeping in her car because of the electrical devices and Wi-Fi in motel rooms. She longed to return home to the Golden State: 'This is a tough place to live,' she said of Green Bank, 'I really don't know how I'm going to support myself.'

Cooney had brought a US $120 million lawsuit against San Diego Gas & Electric and others over the forced installation of smart meters in her previous neighbourhood: 'There was no proper testing on them prior to installation,' she said, 'I've lost my health, my cat, my boyfriend, my home, my money and my business... I might as well fight to get some of it back.'

Nicols Fox had written for the *Economist* on food safety issues for more than a decade and written three books before she sold her house on Maine's Mount Desert Island and moved in 2008 to Renwick, West Virginia, in the Radio Quiet Zone. Fox wasn't given to wild speculation or conspiracy theories, but shooting pains, plummeting heart rates and difficulty speaking, she concluded, were the result of years staring into a computer: 'I got more and more sensitive, and eventually there was a day when my body just screamed when I touched the keyboard.'

In her little house in the Radio Quiet Zone, she wrote on a typewriter and wore a shirt woven with silver fibres to reduce radio frequency exposure. She switched off the electricity whenever possible and used gas lamps. She hadn't left the area in five years.

'I don't care if there's research or not,' she said, 'I've done the research. I've sat in the doctor's office and seen my heart rate drop to 36 beats a minute when they turn the equipment on.'

'Why would I turn my life upside down, abandon my career and sell my house to fake a disease?'

By the summer of 2013, there were 36 electrically hypersensitive people in the Radio Quiet Zone, swelling the population of Green Bank to 147. Some of the locals here and in nearby Marlinton were not happy. There was talk of a threat to rental values and jobs. Diane Schou, after campaigning to turn off the fluorescent lights at the community centre, had had packages stolen from her porch and found a dead groundhog in her mailbox: 'We don't want your kind of people here,' she was told. Deborah Cooney had brought up the issue of microwave radiation at a town meeting and been banned from the radio observatory: she also claimed her tyres had been slashed.

Meanwhile, more people were arriving. Bert Schou was getting calls from folks in New Mexico, Oklahoma, and Virginia, asking if they could come and stay. Diane wanted to raise money to build a resource centre where the hypersensitive could stay and be medically evaluated in a radiation-free setting. Was the scene set for a small town stand-off, or some kind of a return to the community for electromagnetic refugees? The answer was probably both.

*

Deborah Cooney had brought a lawsuit as an individual against the installers of smart meters in California. In Canada, Chief Clarence Louie of the Osoyoos Indian Band was speaking on behalf of a people:

'Thursday, June 13, 2013'

'Native News'

'Nixing Smart Meters'

'Osoyoos Band opts to err on the side of caution.'

'On behalf of the Osoyoos Indian Band, Chief Clarence Louie announced today that he and all Band Council members have signed a governing document prohibiting Fortis BC, the local utility company, from installing Smart Meters on the approximately 703 homes and businesses on the Osoyoos Indian Reserve.'

'Having been presented with science-based evidence, the Band Council and I are convinced that Fortis' proposed wireless smart meters in meshed-grid networks have potential to harm our children and our environment. No scientist on the planet has been able to verify the safety of these extremely dangerous devices that emit microwave radiation 24/7 in perpetuity and which cannot be turned off.'

'As Chief of the Osoyoos Indian band, my first duty is to protect my people, our future generations and our lands. For that reason, the Band Council and I believe we need to err on the side of caution and respect the world's leading independent scientists who say – and have evidence to prove – that electromagnetic radiation, especially pulsed radio and microwave frequency radiation is harmful to all living things.'

'I am proud of our Council for standing up and voting to prohibit the installation of smart meters on our lands in order to protect not only our own people, but all the peoples who reside and work on the Osoyoos Indian Band lands.'

What was it about the technology of 'Smart Meters' that alarmed customers as diverse as Chief Louie, Deborah Cooney and Brian Stein and the Radiation Research Trust?

The 2012 Bioinitiative Report had put it thus:

'A Single Smart Appliance inside a Home Can Produce RF Power Density Levels Shown to Cause Biological Effects.'

'Unfortunately, the problem of excess exposure to RF radiation will get worse as Smart Appliances are adopted. They contain their own internal RF transmitters and receivers. Those Smart Appliances are designed to communicate with Smart Meters and to report through the Smart Meters to the electric power company. The data the Smart Appliances report will be sufficient for the electric power company to identify which appliances you own, when you use them, and how much power they consume, throughout the day and the night. The electric power company may even be able to turn the Smart Appliances off by sending a wireless signal to the Smart Meter that is then transferred to the Smart Appliances, but that is less certain at this time.'

'When these Smart Appliances are installed in a home, they will significantly increase the radiation levels in that home for several reasons:

'They will begin transmitting, and from distances very close to the residents.'

'The number of Smart Appliances in the home may increase with time as the residents gradually replace their old appliances with new Smart Appliances, increasing the total radiation level.'

'The Smart Meters will transmit more frequently, in order to communicate with the Smart Appliances. Even a single Smart Appliance can produce RF power densities of concern.'

'*An inspection of the appended Biological Effects Chart indicates the following:*

'*The power density at 1 meter (3 feet) from a Smart Appliance is higher than the power density that triggered biological effects in 32 of the 67 studies.*'

'*The power density at 3 meters (10 feet) from a Smart Appliance is higher than the power density that triggered biological effects in 21 of the 67 studies.*'

'*The power density at 10 meters (33 feet) from a Smart Appliance is higher than the power density that triggered biological effects in 10 of the 67 studies.*'

'*These observations do not bode well for having 5, 10, or 15 Smart Appliances in a home. The RF radiation from even a few Smart Appliances, because they will be so close to the residents, may rival that of a home's more distant Smart Meter. And the RF radiation from a large number of Smart Appliances may exceed that of a home's Smart Meter.*'

*

In Denmark, the latest industry-funded study refuting the health hazards of mobile phone use had been criticised for its methodology by independent researchers such as Professor Joel Moskowitz, Olle Johannsson and Lennart Hardell.

'*Mobile Phone Use and the Risk of Skin Cancer: A Nationwide Cohort Study in Denmark*'

'*Poulsen AH, Friis S, Johansen C, Jensen A, Frei P, Kjær SK, Dalton SO, Schüz J. Mobile Phone Use and the Risk of Skin Cancer: A Nationwide Cohort Study in Denmark. Am J Epidemiol. 2013 Jun 20. [Epub ahead of print]*'

'*A limitation of our study was the lack of data on the amount of mobile phone use, which prevented us from evaluating potential risks associated with the heaviest use. Also, we had no information on the use of hands-free kits, which reduce exposure to the head and neck, or use of cordless phones, which operate in the same frequency range as mobile phones'.*

'A further limitation was misclassification of exposure. We were unable to identify subscriptions that were not registered in the name of single persons; therefore, subscription holders who did not use their mobile phones would be erroneously classified as exposed, and subjects without a subscription but still using a mobile phone would be erroneously classified as unexposed. This resulted in heavy users on a company contract being classified as non-users. Moreover, subjects who took out their subscriptions after 1995 were classified as unexposed.'

Even the researchers themselves in the Danish study had felt impelled to flag up their misgivings in their 'findings'.

Meanwhile, in the UK, this study was being quoted by the Health Protection Authority (HPA) as the largest and most authoritative of its kind and proof that there was no problem.

*

Elsewhere in Denmark, five North Jutland schoolgirls had reached an independent conclusion:

'Experiments with Cress [and Wi-Fi] in 9th Grade attracts international attention [Denmark] 16th May 2013'

'Researchers from England, Holland and Sweden have shown great interest in the five girls' biology experiments.'

Lea Nielsen, Mathilde Neilsen, Signe Nielsen, Sisse Coltau and Rikke Holm were ninth-graders at Hjallerup School in North Jutland. All the girls had been having difficulty sleeping at night and concentrating during the school day:

'We thought it was because we were sleeping with our mobiles next to our heads,' said Lea Neilsen.

With no equipment at school to test the effects of microwave radiation, the girls created their own experiment. They placed 400 cress seeds in twelve trays and placed the trays in two batches of six in two rooms at the same temperature. All the trays were given the same amount of water and sun over twelve days. One batch of six trays was in a room with no wireless radiation: the other was placed in a room containing two Wi-Fi routers.

Twelve days later, the cress seeds in the Wi-Fi-free trays were growing normally. The cress seeds in the trays exposed to the Wi-Fi routers were not growing normally: some had mutated and some had died: 'Truly frightening,' was Lea Neilsen's verdict,' we were very shocked by the result.'

The Danish media had greeted the recent industry-funded study with headlines such as *'Largest Study Yet – No Risk from Cell Phone Use'*: it congratulated the girls on their findings and the fact that they had secured a place in the 'Young Scientists' competition. Professor Olle Johansson from the Karolinska Institute in Stockholm was similarly impressed: 'The girls stayed within the scope of their knowledge, skilfully implemented and developed a very elegant experiment,' he said, 'The wealth of detail and accuracy is exemplary: choosing cress was very intelligent.'

Professor Johansson planned to replicate the experiment with his colleague Professor Marie-Claire Cammaert at the Free University of Brussels.

Meanwhile, their own lesson was not lost on the five ninth-graders: 'None of us sleeps with the mobile next to the bed any more,' said Lea Neilsen, 'and the computer is always off.'

*

Education and the wellbeing of the next generation were becoming the arenas in which the conflict was played out between industry-funded and independent studies of the effects of microwaves on human beings, living organisms, flora and fauna and the environment.

In India, one of the world's most populous nations with a fast-growing young next generation of producers and consumers, Professor Girish Kumar had witnessed how a Vodafone-sponsored conference could attempt to influence opinion. India was famously corrupt when it came to the protection of commercial interests: yet even one of the world's most powerful companies had failed to convince the Indian Government.

The Department of Telecommunication had already lowered the permissible radiation limit for mobile towers to 0.45 watts per square metre – one hundredth of the ICNIRP guidelines – for Indian mobile operators. The Government had also made it mandatory for the specific absorption rate (SAR) to be displayed on mobile handsets. Imported phones could only be sold in India if the SAR was below 1.6 watts per kilogram, which was lower than the European norms of up to 2 watts.

Now the Indian government was calling for further research:

'NEW DELHI: *Amid concerns over radiation from cell phone towers, government on Friday called for research proposals to study the possible impact of electromagnetic frequency radiation on humans and living organisms.*'

'*The call for proposals by the Science and Engineering Research Board (SERB) comes in the wake of conflicting reports on the impact of cell tower radiation with a section claiming that it caused illness including cancer while others saying that there was no definitive finding to support it.*'

'*The study, to be funded in campaign mode, is a joint initiative supported by the SERB, a statutory body under the Department of Science and Technology, and the Department of Telecommunications.*'

'*The researchers are expected to study the impact of electromagnetic frequency radiation (EMF-r) in the non-ionising band -- 300 MHz to 3 GHz -- on biota and ecology.*'

'*The researchers have been asked to focus on impact of EMF-r on any aspect --physiological, genetic, ecological, growth, development-- at any level including cellular, sub-cellular, molecular, sub-molecular in any model system including humans, plants, animals, birds, fishes and microbes.'*

'Studies on the aspects of epidemiology, social behaviour and safety are also within the ambit of the research.'

'There have been reports in a section of the media about the purported ill-effects of EMF-r from cell towers and mobile handsets.'

*

In Germany, neuroscientist Dr Manfred Spitzer called for digital media to be banned from classrooms before children became 'addicted' and the damage to brain development was irreversible; doctors in South Korea were warning of a surge in 'digital dementia' among young people who had become so reliant on electronic devices that they could no longer remember everyday details like their phone numbers.

South Korea was one of the most digitally dominated nations in the world and the problem of internet addiction among adults and children had been recognised as far back as the late 1990s. The term 'digital dementia' had been coined to describe a deterioration in cognitive abilities more commonly seen in people who had suffered a head injury or psychiatric illness.

"Over-use of smartphones and game devices hampers the balanced development of the brain," Byun Gi-won, a doctor at the Balance Brain Centre in Seoul, told the *JoongAng Daily* newspaper.

'Heavy users are likely to develop the left side of their brains, leaving the right side untapped or underdeveloped,' he said: the right side of the brain being linked with concentration, with failure to develop affecting attention and memory span, which could in as many as 15 per cent of cases lead to the early onset of dementia.

Sufferers were also reported to be experiencing emotional underdevelopment, with children more at risk than adults because their brains were still growing.

More than 67 per cent of South Koreans had a smartphone, the highest in the world, with that figure standing at more than 64 per cent in teenagers, up from 21.4 per cent in 2011, according to the Ministry of Science, ICT and Future Planning. The percentage of people aged between 10 and 19 who used their smartphones for more than seven hours every day had leapt to 18.4 per cent, an increase of seven per cent from the previous year.

'Kim Min-woo, 15, started having memory problems recently. He started flunking tests in subjects that required heavy bouts of memorization. And then he couldn't remember the six-digit keypad code to get into his own home. He had to call the code up on his smartphone to get in the door.'

'Kim's mother took him to a doctor and the diagnosis was shocking: Kim had symptoms of early onset dementia due to intense exposure to digital technology. Since the age of five, Kim was tethered to either the television or the computer. He is an avid computer game lover.'

'His brain's ability to transfer information to long-term memory has been impaired because of his heavy exposure to digital gadgets,' said psychiatrist Kim Dae-jin at Seoul St. Mary's Hospital in southern Seoul, who diagnosed Kim and is treating him...'

*

In Orange County, the third most populous county in California, USA, in the summer of 2013, the media started carrying stories about possible links between microwave emissions and Orange County as the 'Autism capital of the state'. In Connecticut, stories began to appear about scientists from Yale, Albany and Columbia Universities warning a symposium in Stonington of 'a grave public health danger that is being obscured by corporate interests'.

In Israel, as a result of a report by attorney Dafna Tachover, the Supreme Court ordered the Government to investigate the number of children suffering from electrohypersensitivity.

Research carried out by neuroscientists at Laurentian University and Cambrian College of Applied Arts and Technology in Ontario, Canada, had already concluded that exposure to pulsed magnetic fields could permanently alter the blood chemistry and brain development in male and female albino Wistar rats. In Toronto, the Elementary Teachers Federation of Ontario was holding its annual general meeting.

The EFTA was Canada's largest teaching union, represented 76,000 teachers in the province. On 15 August, 2013, the vote was carried that pupils' cell phones should be switched off and stored away during school hours. This was one of a series of motions proposing that cell phone radiation be acknowledged as a workplace hazard. Another motion requested that school boards no longer conceal Wi-Fi transmitters in ceilings, and include them in a hazard control programme.

'There is cause for concern for members' health and safety, especially women,' said Sandra Walsh, representing Peel District at the meeting.

Less than a month earlier, in Ottawa, the chairman of Canadians For Safe Technology (C4ST), Daniel Krewski, had been forced to resign over conflicts of interest from a panel examining safety level for cell towers, cell phones and Wi-Fi in Canada.

Mr Krewski was also a member of the Mclaughlin Institute for Public Health, which was founded and part-funded by the Canadian Wireless Industry Association: he had neglected to mention that, while reviewing Canada's Safety Code, he had accepted a $126,000 contract 'to convince an unwilling Canadian public' that cell towers were safe.

The panel had been chosen by the Royal Society of Canada. The new C4ST chairman, Frank Clegg, had been President of Microsoft Canada for fourteen years before committing himself to campaigning for safer wireless technology: he wanted another scientist with close mobile industry ties, John Moulder, removed from the panel: 'Mr Moulder is an American industry consultant,' said Clegg, 'he has no place influencing Canada's safety review.'

In the United States, the President of the American Academy of Paediatrics, which represented 60,000 health professionals, wrote a letter to the Acting Commissioner of the Federal Communications Commission (FCC) and the Commissioner of the US Food and Drug Administration (FDA). He urged the FCC and FDA to adopt electromagnetic radiation safety standards that reflected current use:

'August 29, 2013'

'Dear Acting Chairwoman Clyburn and Commissioner Hamburg:'

'The American Academy of Pediatrics (AAP), a non-profit professional organization of 60,000 primary care pediatricians, pediatric medical subspecialists, and pediatric surgical specialists dedicated to the health, safety and well-being of infants, children, adolescents, and young adults appreciates this opportunity to comment on the Proposed Rule "Reassessment of Exposure to Radiofrequency Electromagnetic Fields Limits and Policies" published in the Federal Register on June 4, 2013.'

'In the past few years, a number of American and international health and scientific bodies have contributed to the debate over cell phone radiation and its possible link to cancer. The International Agency for Research on Cancer (IARC), part of the United Nations' World Health Organization, said in June 2011 that a family of frequencies that includes mobile phone emissions is "possibly carcinogenic to humans." The National Cancer Institute has stated that although studies have not demonstrated that RF energy from cell phones definitively causes cancer, more research is needed because cell phone technology and cell phone use are changing rapidly. These studies and others clearly demonstrate the need for further research into this area and highlight the importance of reassessing current policy to determine if it is adequately protective of human health.'

'As radiation standards are reassessed, the AAP urges the FCC to adopt radiation standards that:

'*Protect children's health and well-being. Children are not little adults and are disproportionately impacted by all environmental exposures, including cell phone radiation. Current FCC standards do not account for the unique vulnerability and use patterns specific to pregnant women and children. It is essential that any new standard for cell phones or other wireless devices be based on protecting the youngest and most vulnerable populations to ensure they are safeguarded throughout their lifetimes.*'

'*Reflect current use patterns. The FCC has not assessed the standard for cell phone radiation since 1996. Approximately 44 million people had mobile phones when the standard was set; today, there are more than 300 million mobile phones in use in the United States. While the prevalence of wireless phones and other devices has skyrocketed, the behaviors around cell phone uses have changed as well. The number of mobile phone calls per day, the length of each call, and the amount of time people use mobile phones has increased, while cell phone and wireless technology has undergone substantial changes. Many children, adolescents and young adults, now use cell phones as their only phone line and they begin using wireless phones at much younger ages.*'

'*Pregnant women may carry their phones for many hours per day in a pocket that keeps the phone close to their uterus. Children born today will experience a longer period of exposure to radio-frequency fields from cellular phone use than will adults, because they start using cellular phones at earlier ages and will have longer lifetime exposures. FCC regulations should reflect how people are using their phones today.*'

'*Provide meaningful consumer disclosure. The FCC has noted that it does not provide consumers with sufficient information about the RF exposure profile of individual phones to allow consumers to make informed purchasing decisions. The current metric of RF exposure available to consumers, the Specific Absorption Rate, is not an accurate predictor of actual exposure.*'

'*AAP is supportive of FCC developing standards that provide consumers with the information they need to make informed choices in selecting mobile phone purchases, and to help parents to better understand any potential risks for their children. To that end, we support the use of metrics that are specific to the exposure children will experience.'*

'The AAP supports the reassessment of radiation standards for cell phones and other wireless products and the adoption of standards that are protective of children and reflect current use patterns. If you have questions, please contact Clara Filice in the AAP's Washington Office at 202/347-8600.'
'Sincerely,'
'Thomas K. McInerny, MD FAAP'
'President'

'Letter sent to:'

'The Honorable Mignon L. Clyburn
Acting Commissioner
Federal Communications Commission
445 12th Street SW
Washington, DC 20054'

'The Honorable Dr. Margaret A. Hamburg
Commissioner
U.S. Food and Drug Administration
10903 New Hampshire Avenue
Silver Spring, MD 20993'

*

The combination of American trades unions, public bodies of teachers and health professionals and the litigious potential of the American consumer, was beginning to make the WHO's reclassification of EMFs as a potential B2 carcinogen look less an alarmist gesture than an understatement.

'Four case studies of young women with breast cancer who kept cell phones in their bras.'

'John G. West, 'Multifocal Breast Cancer in Young Women with Prolonged Contact between Their Breasts and Their Cellular Phones,' Case Reports in Medicine, vol. 2013, Article ID 354682, 5 pages, 2013. doi:10.1155/2013/354682.'

'Today, a peer-reviewed publication appears in Case Reports in Medicine by six physicians that discusses four such cases.'

'John G. West, Nimmi S. Kapoor, Shu-Yuan Liao, June W. Chen, Lisa Bailey, and Robert A. Nagourney. Multifocal Breast Cancer in Young Women with Prolonged Contact between Their Breasts and Their Cellular Phones. Case Reports in Medicine. 2013.'

'Breast cancer occurring in women under the age of 40 is uncommon in the absence of family history or genetic predisposition, and prompts the exploration of other possible exposures or environmental risks.'

'This paper discusses a case series of four young women—ages from 21 to 39—with multifocal invasive breast cancer that raises the concern of a possible association with electromagnetic field exposures from cell phones. All patients regularly carried their cell phones directly against their breasts in their brassieres for up to 10 hours a day, for several years, and developed tumors in areas of their breasts immediately underlying the phones. All patients had no family history of breast cancer, tested negative for BRCA1 and BRCA2, and had no other known breast cancer risks.'

'Their breast imaging is reviewed, showing clustering of multiple tumor foci in the breast directly under the area of phone contact. Pathology of all four cases shows striking similarity; all tumors are hormone-positive, low-intermediate grade, having an extensive intraductal component, and all tumors have near identical morphology.'

'These cases raise awareness to the lack of safety data of prolonged direct contact with cellular phones.'

'Of particular note' ... the effect of EMR on children can be several times higher than that of adults. It is possible that the growing, dividing breast tissue that occurs during puberty may be particularly vulnerable to cellular phone EMR, accounting in part for at least two of the cases reported here.'

*

Peer-reviewed publications such as this in *Case Reports in Medicine* countered mobile industry criticism that lack of peer reviews constituted 'bad' science. With Orange County being claimed as the 'autism capital of the USA', two further peer-reviewed papers were published in *Pathophysiology* in the autumn of 2013 pointing to the increased incidence of autism in American children, an increase highlighted by Cindy Sage and Dr Martha Herbert of the Harvard School of Medicine in the 2012 *Bioinitiative Report*.

In 1975, one child in 5,000 had been diagnosed autistic: in 2013, the figure was one child in 88, or one child in 50 according to 2012 estimates that included the eight-year-old and younger cohort.

The reputed annual cost to the taxpayer - US $137 billion – was nearly as high as the EU annual cost for cancer. As Cindy Sage pointed out, this increase in diagnosed autism paralleled the explosive rise in wireless technologies and pulsed radio frequency radiation.

*

In the USA, while the cell phone industry was facing the first class actions from brain tumour sufferers and their families, the government was still trying to conceal or rewrite the history of the effects of microwave radiation and EMFs during the Cold War.

The people of California were rejecting the installation of smart meters, Orange County was being cited as the microwave-driven 'autism centre of America' and ES 'refugees' like Bert and Diane Schou were relocating to places such as the Radio Quiet Zone in Green Bank, Virginia.

In India, both the State of Rajasthan and the City of Mumbai had passed laws prohibiting the installation of microwave masts on the roofs of hospitals and schools and in playgrounds because they were 'hazardous to life.' Indian safety thresholds were already lower than those of ICNIRP, but when scientists at the Netaji Subhas Chandra Bose Cancer Research Institute (NSCRI) studied 200 people living in an area of high density mobile towers in central Kolkata, within a fifty metre radius of the towers they found widespread physiological dysfunction.

Around 70% of residents suffered from fatigue: 30% had partial loss of memory; 20% had dizziness and 25% had sleeping disorders. While 20% had skin infections, around 12-15% had hearing impairment and 10% suffered from cardiac problems. Almost half those surveyed said they had difficulty in concentrating and 30% said they were irritable. Two babies born in the previous six months had congenital defects.

'Interestingly, most of the subjects of the study said the intensity of their ailments goes down once they leave their homes and reverts to the earlier stage once they return,' said Ashish Mukhopadhyay of NSCRI, 'While we need further evidence, this is something that technical experts should worry about.'

'We already have level 1 evidence to prove that those who live near towers and are exposed to this radiation 24 hours a day are not safe. It is quite possible for them to suffer from disorders, especially hearing impairment, visual problems and loss of memory. There is as yet no direct evidence to show that tower radiation causes cancer. But we need more studies to check whether brain tumours are related to this,' said Jaydip Biswas, director, Chittaranjan National Cancer Research Institute (CNCRI).

Biswas added that even without such evidence, towers should not be allowed in congested neighbourhoods and near schools.

In Russia, Professor Yury Grigoriev joined the ranks of world-class independent scientists warning of the health risks from radio frequency radiation. In China, microwave masts were removed from a university in Hong Kong. In Belgium, the sale of mobile phones was forbidden to children under the age of seven; in France, nurseries and elementary schools were being hardwired and declared Wi-Fi-free zones, vindicating the warnings issued in Germany by neuroscientist Dr Manfred Spitzer.

In South Korea, research linked the use of mobile phones by children and teenagers with 'digital dementia'. In Italy, the courts had found in favour of Innocenzo Marcolini on the basis of independent research by Professor Lennart Hardell.

In Denmark, schoolgirls were proving that Wi-Fi routers mutated and killed cress seeds: similar effects on insect life were being noted by Professor Margaritis and his colleagues in Greece.

In Australia, a court had recognised electrohypersensitivity and found in favour of Dr MacDonald; a Sydney University Physics lecturer Dr James McCaughan resigned after suffering ill-effects he believed were due to the presence of smartphones in the lecture room. Dr Marie-Therese Gibson resigned after nineteen years as Principal of the exclusive Tangara School for Girls due to health problems she attributed to Wi-Fi routers: 'I gave the best part of my life to that school, but I had to resign because I couldn't exist in that environment," she said, 'I realised as time went on I was getting sicker and sicker and couldn't sleep at night. There were parts of the school I just couldn't go into.'

'I started getting strange headaches and tremendous fatigue, and I found I couldn't think clearly. My thyroid is kaput and my body can't make melatonin."

'Why should students be immersed in it for six or seven hours a day when they're (only) using it for one?" she went on, 'It just doesn't make sense to me.'

In Canada, Chief Clarence Louie and the Osoyoos Indian band were rejecting the installation of smart meters and the Saanich District School Board on Vancouver Island had banned Wi-Fi in elementary schools due to the uncertainty around children's health. Also in British Columbia, the Kootenay Lakes school district voted to maintain one school without Wi-Fi in order to provide a safe haven for students sensitive to microwave radiation.

In Bermuda, the Bermuda Re insurance company refused to underwrite any more policies indemnifying mobile phone companies against lawsuits alleging health damage from users. In the spring of 2014, another major insurance firm, Swiss Re also issued a warning about large losses from 'unforeseen consequences' of radio frequency radiation.

In France, videos were aired across TV and social media showing the realities of the lives of electrorefugees, with testimony from independent scientists and researchers including Professor Dariusz Leszczynski and Louis Slesin.

Were all these the responses to 'psychological' reactions? In rats, unborn and adult, and plants, as well as children and adults – and insurers?

In Athens, from 27-28 March, 2014, the European Commission and the Greek Atomic Energy Commission held a two-day workshop on the health effects of electromagnetic fields: delegates included representatives of the EU, World Health Organisation, mobile phone operators and academia.

The event was also the launch of the Scientific Committee on Emerging and Newly Identified Health Risks (SCENIHR) draft opinion on the potential health effects of electromagnetic fields. SCNIHR's findings would influence the European United and European Parliament: both bodies which had been criticised for their lack of action in this matter by Professor Yury Grigoriev and others.

MEP Marian Harkin opened the Athens event by reminding delegates that 500 million citizens were relying on SCENIHR's findings. Among these EU citizens and delegates present were Eileen O'Connor of the UK Radiation Research Trust and former rocket scientist Sissel Halmoy of the International EMF Alliance. Both were to be disappointed in their expectations: specifically by the exclusion from the SCENIHR findings of the work of Professor Lennart Hardell.

The five Hardell papers excluded by SCENIHR were the first to correlate mobile phone usage with incidences of brain tumours over a 20-year period, longer than any other epidemiological studies. They found a clear correlation between mobile phone usage and two types of brain tumours, acoustic neuromas and the deadliest of all brain cancers, gliomas.

Yet, the Hardell scenario was not only excluded, but denigrated by members of SCENIHR such as Joachim Schüz, Head of IARC's Section of Environment and Radiation, who also promoted the controversial Danish study while criticising Hardell's publications, and by Paolo Rossi, of the Italian Ministry of Health.

Rossi conceded that 'Children should not use mobile phones as a toy', but then criticised the decision from the Italian supreme court judge for awarding compensation in the Marcolini case, a judgement which had found in favour of Hardell's findings over those of ICIRP.

Eileen O'Connor held up the five Hardell papers missing from SCENIHR's report for all to see and called for them to be included within the SCENIHR review. She also read aloud from the conclusion from one of the papers: 'I was hoping for an equal and honest debate to be held in Athens,' O'Connor reflected, 'but was sadly surprised and extremely disappointed by the lack of inclusion for stakeholders with alternative views to scientists representing SCENIHR in Athens. I was one of only two voices invited to present with an alternative view and had taken time to prepare a presentation in the hope and anticipation of receiving a warm welcome and equal opportunity to be heard and taken seriously.'

Sissel Halmøy agreed. This was the 'good and bad scientists' industry lobby at work when the greater interests of the citizen were at stake:

'It was plain for all to see that there was clear selection bias from SCENIHR's review as they clearly cherry picked their own research and promoted it as gold standard while heavily criticising Lennart Hardell's research.'

'This issue needs to be addressed and dealt with as a matter of global urgency,' she said, 'Our European Community is being irradiated by microwaves, people are becoming ill, and the World Health Organization has declared a possible correlation to cancer in humans. It's not rocket science. It's just common sense and sound science.'

Halmøy's presentation had highlighted criticisms of the SCENIHR document by former *New York Times* science writer Blake Levitt and University of Washington's Dr Henry Lai, the latter like Lennart Hardell regarded by many as a 'gold standard' scientist.

Lai and Levitt said the report failed to do a thorough review of recent literature on non-ionizing electromagnetic fields (EMF) and biological health effects. Only selected papers had been evaluated using ambiguous criteria.

'It is outrageous,' Lai and Levitt continued, 'to ignore any effect of EMF exposure on human health and a crime to humanity not to recommend any action to curtail the exposure.'

Post-Athens, calls were immediately made for the report to be returned for a new evaluation, and for independent experts such as Hardell and Lai to be included within SCENIHR: in accordance with the spirit of the event as expressed in the opening address, which had stressed the need for inclusivity and transparency.

Eileen O'Connor said she was putting those at the conference 'on notice': 'As of March 28, 2014, representatives of the telecom industry, government officials, and WHO scientists absolutely, irrefutably have the latest science from Hardell and know that

Hardell himself is calling for RF to be classified a Group 1 carcinogen.'

'The clock has now started ticking on liability,' she concluded, 'No more excuses. SCENIHR, the industry, the EU Commission and WHO are now fully informed.'

All four of them, it seemed, were increasingly out of step with the thinking on the physiological effects of electromagnetic fields and radio frequency radiation of the Swedish, French and Belgian governments, the Italian, Australian and Russian courts, and two of the world's largest insurance companies.

'Is Wi-Fi killing us...slowly?' asked Mark Gibbs in **Network World**, Aug 21, 2014.

'What would it take to get you to not use Wi-Fi? I don't mean simply not connecting to it; I mean not having Wi-Fi switched on. At all. And what about cell phones? I know that the issue of cell phone safety has come and gone and most authorities have dismissed the risks as negligible. But what if the risks to you are trivial, but not to your children?'

'Human-generated Electro Magnetic Radiation (EMR) in the general environment was negligible at the beginning of the Twentieth Century, but by 1933 the problem of Electro Magnetic Interference (EMI) was becoming significant. In that year, the International Electrotechnical Commission in Paris "recommended the International Special Committee on Radio Interference (CISPR) be set up to deal with the emerging problem of EMI."

'Since then, despite much legislation and regulation, the general EMR background has increased significantly in the Western hemisphere and even more dramatically in suburban and urban areas, with radio and television being among the greatest contributors. That said, the general suburban and urban EMR levels are to the order of few tens of $\mu W/m^2$ which has been thought to be a harmless level of exposure.'

Gibbs cited the paper, *'Why children absorb more microwave radiation than adults: The consequences'*, published in June 2014.

The authors, L. Lloyd Morgan, Santosh Kesari and Devra Lee Davis summarized how they used computer simulation based on MRI scans of children to model microwave absorption and found:

'Children absorb more microwave radiation (MWR) than adults because their brain tissues are more absorbent, their skulls are thinner and their relative size is smaller. Microwave radiation from wireless devices has been declared a possible human carcinogen. Children are at greater risk than adults when exposed to any carcinogen.'

'The problem is that the consequences of exposure are anything but immediate:'

'Because the average latency time between first exposure and diagnosis of a tumor can be decades, tumors induced in children may not be diagnosed until well into adulthood. The fetus is particularly vulnerable to MWR. MWR exposure can result in degeneration of the protective myelin sheath that surrounds brain neurons.'

'And, of course, the explosion of radio-controlled toys has an effect:'

'MWR-emitting toys are being sold for use by young infants and toddlers. Digital dementia has been reported in school age children. A case study has shown when cell phones are placed in teenage girls' bras multiple primary breast cancers develop beneath where the phones are placed.'

'So, what are we going to do? Here's some compelling evidence that MWR presents a real risk, yet we currently live in a society flooded with microwave radio signals and that situation is only going to become even more pronounced. The paper points out that:'

'MWR exposure limits have remained unchanged for 19 years. All manufacturers of smartphones have warnings which describe the minimum distance at which phone must be kept away from users in order to not exceed the present legal limits for exposure to

MWR. The exposure limit for laptop computers and tablets is set when devices are tested 20 cm away from the body. Belgium, France, India and other technologically sophisticated governments are passing laws and/or issuing warnings about children's use of wireless devices.'

'Laws and warnings are all very well but it's pretty much certain that all restrictions on products that use microwave technology will err on the safe side; that is, the side that's safe for industry, not the side of what's safe for society.'

'Will we look back (sadly) in fifty or a hundred years and marvel at how Wi-Fi and cell phones were responsible for the biggest health crisis in human history?'

*

In the autumn of 2014 the translation appeared of the following article from the Finnish newspaper *Satakunnan kansa*:

Bombshell: Former Nokia Chief Technologist says mobile phones wrecked his health.

'Former Nokia Boss: Mobile Phones wrecked my health'

'By Anne Nikka'

'[English translation Henrik Eiriksson]'

'Nokia's former Technology Chief, Matti Niemelä, was involved in the development the world's first mobile phones, but fell seriously ill himself from mobile 'phone microwave radiation.'

'In addition, he was diagnosed with Multiple Sclerosis (MS). Some studies suggest that radiation may increase the risk of even MS.'

* * * * * * * * * * * *

'For Tampere-based Matti Niemelä, age 44, life was like in the movies when he as a young man was recruited to work for Nokia

in 1997. The brilliant young man quickly advanced to become Nokia's Chief Technology Officer for ten years, and was involved in developing the world's first mobile phones, memory sticks and WLAN [Wi-Fi] connections.'

'In 2007, Niemelä's career hit a brick wall as his health finally failed. Today, he is only able to move using a walker. Niemelä refuses to use a wheelchair.'

'The irony of this is that I'm no longer able to use any of those devices that I had been developing,' Niemelä says with a smile.'

'Niemelä is one of the unfortunate who have experienced severe symptoms of radiation: 'Traveling around the world with a communicator [early model smartphone] in hand, exposure to radiation was very strong from morning to night, and even at night.'

'Few people have had such an overload of radiation as me,' says Niemelä.'

'The first symptoms appeared already within a year of his employment at Nokia:'

'I was playing badminton, and I could no longer hit the shuttlecock during a serve, even though I'd played badminton for a while.'

'At first Niemelä didn't dare go to the doctor, mainly because of the fear of brain cancer.'

'The symptoms got worse year by year: 'I couldn't walk around while talking on the mobile phone, because it caused coordination problems.' The more intense the exposure, the more his speech slurred.'

'Also my ear felt hot when I talked on the phone for a longer times. I struggled on, using the phone until I could no longer feel my own skin. Then I had to go to the doctor,' Niemelä explains.'

'In 2001, MRI images, and cerebrospinal fluid samples revealed the brutal truth: multiple sclerosis: 'I was kind of relieved, because one can cope with MS, but not so with brain cancer.'

'According to Niemelä, medical representatives aren't willing to take a position on whether mobile phone radiation caused the MS. Preliminary results, however, show that radiation increases the risk of multiple sclerosis.'

'I am a layman, not a doctor. MS is certainly caused by a number of factors, not just mobile phone radiation. The radiation does, however, increase my MS symptoms.'

'Also, symptoms of the disease may easily be confused with the mobile phone radiation symptoms,' Niemelä explains. During the interview, Niemelä's voice begins to slur badly.'

'A sign in the hallway asks you to switch off the mobile 'phone. Even a small radiation exposure is too much: 'I can no longer go to the cinema or stay in public areas with lots of radiation for long. I have not been anywhere for a long time,' says Niemelä who in his forties, must accept that the four walls of his home are now a prison.'

'Although Niemelä has lost his health, career and more recently his marriage, he does not blame anyone: 'I'm not bitter, it was my own choice to work for Nokia.'

'He also doesn't want to scare too many about cell phone dangers: 'A healthy person can use a mobile phone responsibly.'

'Niemelä admits that going public with his story carries a big risk: ' I'm scared to talk about this in public, because I do not want to be labelled as crazy.'

'Niemelä explains that the subject of mobile phone radiation has always been kept silent at Nokia: 'You couldn't talk about it within the company. Yet, among the staff, it was speculated whether the radiation could cause damage. However, no one dared to bring it up, because it could get them fired.'

'Niemelä says he brought up the matter with the doctor for the first time in 2006: 'The doctor told me about a number of patients who are suffering from the same symptoms as me,' Niemelä reveals.'

'Niemelä is particularly concerned about children and their mobile phone use, because the continuous exposure to the ear and head does not do any good:'

'These things have been kept silent for too long. I hope it will become possible to discuss the symptoms openly, and without fear.'

****

'Mobile phone manufacturer Nokia and Microsoft's current Senior Vice President Tom Kuuppelomäki assures that all products meet the requirements set by international health bodies and standards: 'Product safety is of paramount importance both for Nokia and Microsoft.'

'With plenty of Nokia employees using mobile phones during the past decades, wouldn't it have been evident if the radiation was causing symptoms?'

'The World Health Organization has looked at a number of studies, from the last two decades, with the aim to determine whether mobile phones pose a potential health risk.'

'Kuuppelomäki insists that to date, studies have not demonstrated adverse health effects from mobile phone use.'

'What kind of studies on radiation has Nokia done and commissioned since the late 1980s?'

'Nokia and Microsoft are now participating in the MMF (Mobile Manufacturers Forum) research funding, mainly in conjunction with governmental organizations and other industry representatives of the funded research programs.'

'We believe that nonpartisan research will produce the best consumer information on equipment safety.'

'How will the health effects be studied in the future?'

'WHO has made recommendations for further research on electromagnetic fields to enable a thorough risk assessment.'

*

In South Africa, The Cancer Association of South Africa (Cansa) issued a warning that giving children cell phones and other wireless technology devices carried 'enormous' risks.

'Cell phones fry young brains'

'Tanya Farber | 11 December, 2014 00:39'

'Their skulls and brains are still developing and the radiation from cell phones practically 'cooks' their brains," said Professor Michael Herbst, head of health at Cansa.'

'A child's brain is cased in a thinner skull and absorbs more radiation than that of an adult.'

'Dr Devra Davis, president of Environmental Health Trust, a group of global epidemiologists, said: "Retailers are going all out to make devices affordable, and parents are clamouring to buy them. But the standards are based on old models and old assumptions about how we use them."'

'Studies in Europe found the bone marrow of a child's head absorbs 10 times more radiation than that of an adult, while the brain tissue absorbs twice as much.'

'These warnings from [the health trust] are supported by Cansa,' says Herbst, 'The South African public is totally involved with technology but do not seem to be aware of the inherent dangers.'

'iPads, for example, contain radiating antennae that should not be held directly on the body, but children's arms are not long enough to create the distance. Babies play with cell phones, and mothers speak on the devices while breastfeeding.'

'Because of the lag between exposure and disease, said Herbst and Davis, the risks are not taken seriously enough.'

'We may definitely see an increase in the incidence of brain disease in the future,' said Herbst.'

*

In the United States, *Forbes* magazine took up the issue:

'Study Suggests Wi-Fi Exposure More Dangerous To Kids Than Previously Thought'

'Robert J. Szczerba, *Forbes*, Jan 12, 2015'

'Most parents would be concerned if their children had significant exposure to lead, chloroform, gasoline fumes, or the pesticide DDT. The International Agency for Research on Cancer (IRIC), part of the United Nations' World Health Organization (WHO), classifies these and more than 250 other agents as Class 2B Carcinogens. Another entry on that same list is radiofrequency electromagnetic fields (RF/EMF). The main sources of RF/EMF are radios, televisions, microwave ovens, cell phones, and Wi-Fi devices.'

'Uh-oh. Not another diatribe about the dangers of our modern communication systems? Obviously, these devices and the resulting fields are extremely (and increasingly) common in modern society. Even if we want to, we can't eliminate our exposure, or our children's, to RF/EMF. But, we may need to limit that exposure, when possible.'

'That was among the conclusions of a report published in the Journal of Microscopy and Ultrastructure *entitled "Why children absorb more microwave radiation than adults: The consequences." From an analysis of peer-reviewed studies, the authors argue that children and adolescents are at considerable risk from devices that radiate microwaves (and that adults are at a lower, but still significant, risk). The following points were made:'*

'Children absorb a greater amount of microwave radiation than adults.'

'Fetuses are even more vulnerable than children. Therefore pregnant women should avoid exposing their fetus to microwave radiation.'

'Adolescent girls and women should not place cell phones in their bras or in hijabs (headscarf).'

'Cell phone manual warnings make clear an overexposure problem exists.'

'Government warnings have been issued but most of the public are unaware of such warnings.'

'Current exposure limits are inadequate and should be revised.'

'Wireless devices are radio transmitters, not toys. Selling toys that use them should be monitored more closely, or possibly even banned.'

'Children and fetuses absorb more microwave radiation, according to the authors, because their bodies are relatively smaller, their skulls are thinner, and their brain tissue is more absorbent.'

'More generally, the studies cited in the paper found RF/EMF exposure is linked to cancers of the brain and salivary glands, ADHD, low sperm count, and, among girls who keep cell phones in their bra, breast cancer. They also noted that the average time between exposure to a carcinogen and a resultant tumor is three or more decades.'

'Hopefully, more longitudinal studies will be done to verify or contradict the findings so far. In the meantime, are the government's current regulations adequate? The exposure levels they warn against haven't seem to have been updated for more than 19 years.'

'In a Network World opinion article ominously titled "Is Wi-Fi killing us...slowly?" columnist Mark Gibbs makes the point that "... laws and warnings are all very well but it's pretty much certain that all restrictions on products that use microwave technology will err on the safe side; that is, the side that's safe for industry, not the side of what's safe for society." Gibbs then added this ominous closing question, "Will we look back (sadly) in fifty or a hundred years and marvel at how Wi-Fi and cell phones were responsible for the biggest health crisis in human history?"

'But, short of that worst-case scenario, the topic certainly merits more scrutiny, and perhaps some common sense limits on what devices our children use, and for how long.'

*

In Britain, in spite of the rising tide of scientific, consumer and legislative action from around the world lapping at the shores of those islands, the UK Health Protection Agency's successor Public Health England continued to reject the precautionary principle and assert the safety thresholds set by ICNIRP.

At Kings College London, Dr James Rubin continued to address the effects of electromagnetic fields on the biology of humans and animals via the 'psychological' approach. Scientific research by Professor Andrew Goldsworthy, Professor Denis Henshaw and Dr Gerard Hyland into the physiological effects of EMFs and radio frequency radiation in Britain had all but been closed down, 'psychological' clinical trials that had taken place such as those at Essex University were methodologically questionable and the subject – with a few exceptions including those detailed here - was barely mentioned.

When it came to the physiological effects of microwave radiation and electromagnetic fields on human beings and animals, on every aspect of the environment in general, a government charged with a duty of care to its citizens and taxpayers continued to bow unilaterally to the free market and auction 4G bandwidth to the mobile phone industry – trading health for wealth - and, when challenged on the matter, invoked the 'need to know' posture of generations of British government scientists, with the line that 'we know best'.

In Britain, schools were routinely and non-consensually Wi-Fi'd, and five-year-old-children could buy or be bought mobile phones. One in ten five-year-olds owned one, and reports suggested that in addition to 'ensuring' the child's safety, the devices were bought to distract them on long journeys and to stop them from commandeering their parents' phones.

The situation of the UK was increasingly at odds with the growing body of research around the world suggesting that mobile phones and Wi-Fi were causing physiological damage in human beings ranging from ADHD, allergies, autism, Alzheimer's Disease, brain tumours, 'digital dementia' and sleeplessness in teenagers, damage to the blood-brain barrier in children under the age of eighteen, infertility, the ante-natal welfare of foetuses and pregnant mothers, premature ageing and changes in the DNA of humans and animal species.

Only a hitherto small and fractious group of people – the 'ES Community' – were campaigning to raise the issue in the UK to the level of other countries that had already determined they should set their wireless and EMF safety thresholds far below those promoted by ICNIRP.

In Brian Stein's opinion, as far as the British Government and UK Health Protection Agency were concerned: *'This was up there with the Hillsborough football disaster, Lance Armstrong the drug cheat and Jimmy Saville the paedophile - the lone voice versus the authorities in denial. The evidence was there – it just wasn't PC to look at it correctly.'*

But this community was already bigger than its members realised: and it was beginning to join up and organise with the growing body of opinion around the world.

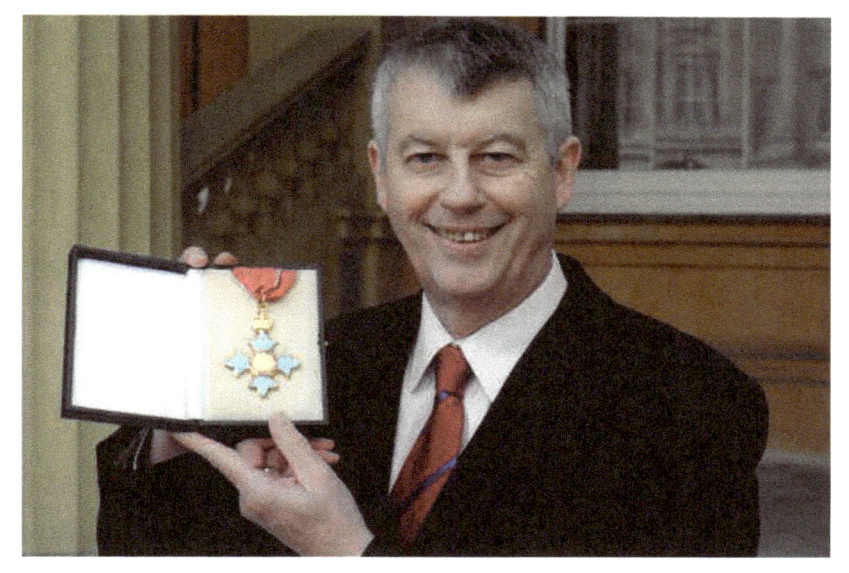

Brian Stein CBE outside Buckingham Palace. *(Brian Stein)*

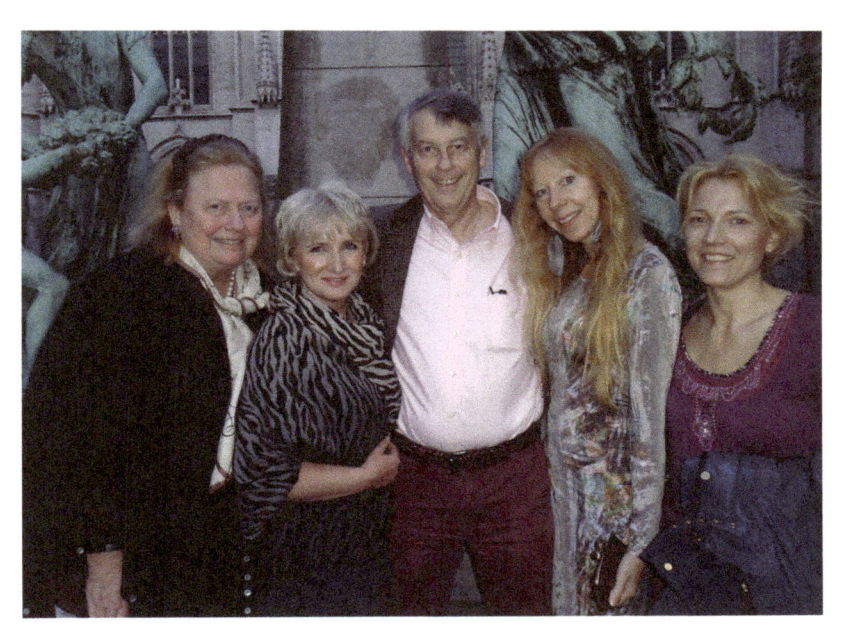

Camilla Rees, Eileen O'Connor, Brian Stein, Dr Erica Mallery-Blythe and Malin Tornqvist at Academie royale de Medecine de Belgique in Brussels. *(Radiation Research Trust)*

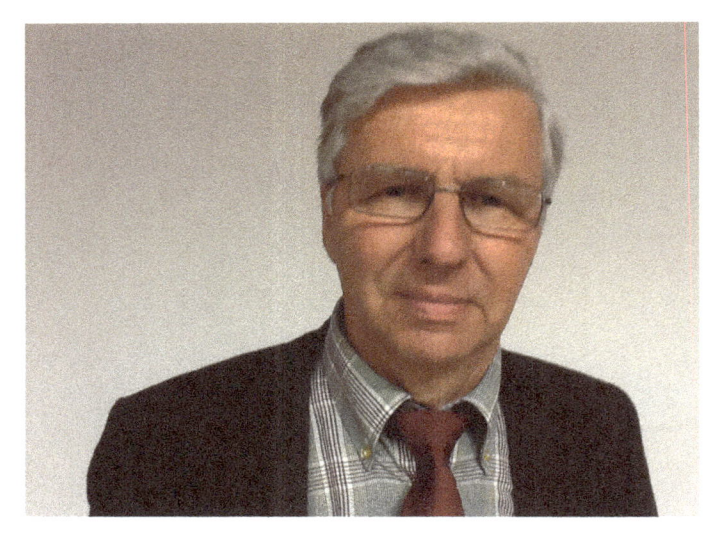

Professor Lennart Hardell, the most respected and widely-cited independent researcher into the damaging health effects of EMFs of his generation. *(Radiation Research Trust)*

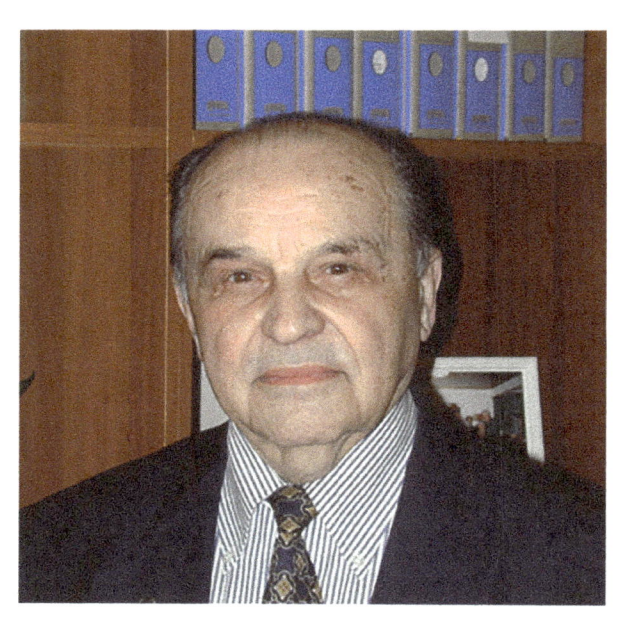

Professor Yury Grigoriev, doyen of Soviet and Russian scientists and leading proponent of the need for greater measures to protect the environment from EMFs. *(Professor Yury Grigoriev)*

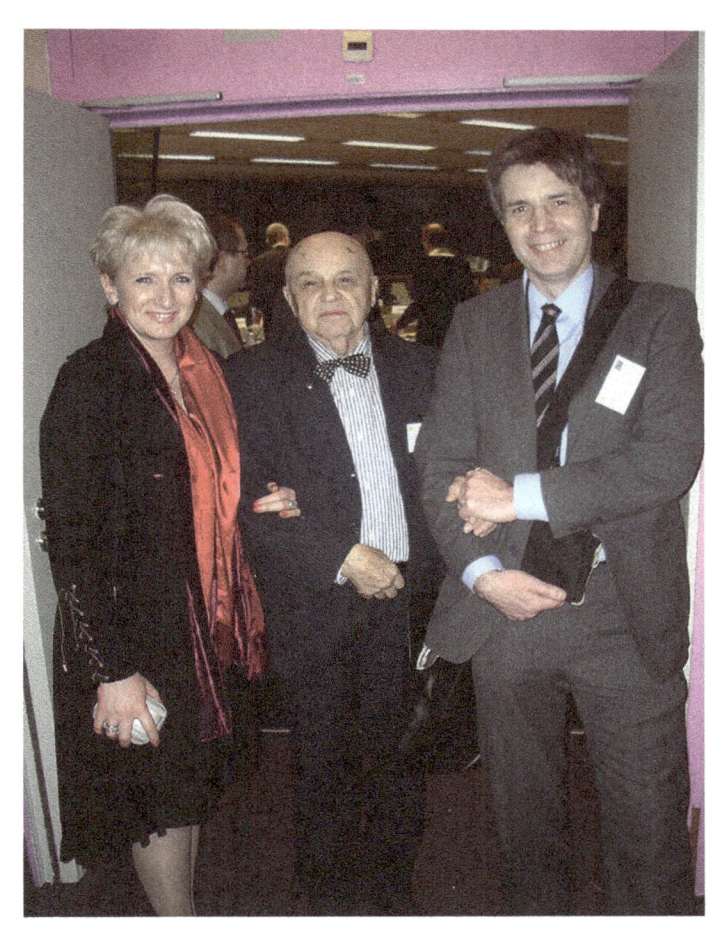

Professor Yury Grigoriev, Eileen O'Connor and Dr Isaac Jamieson of Radiation Research Trust in Brussels. *(Radiation Research Trust)*

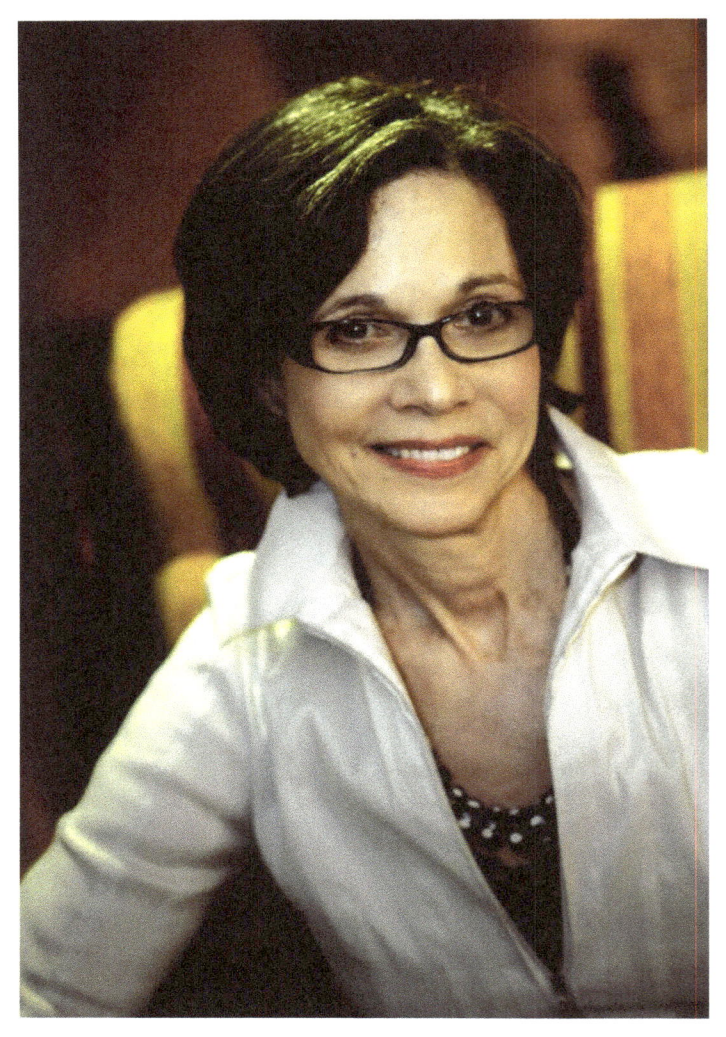

Dr Devra Davis, founder and leader of the Environmental Health Trust (EHT) and America's leading campaigner against the hazards of wireless radiation to babies and children. *(Radiation Research Trust)*

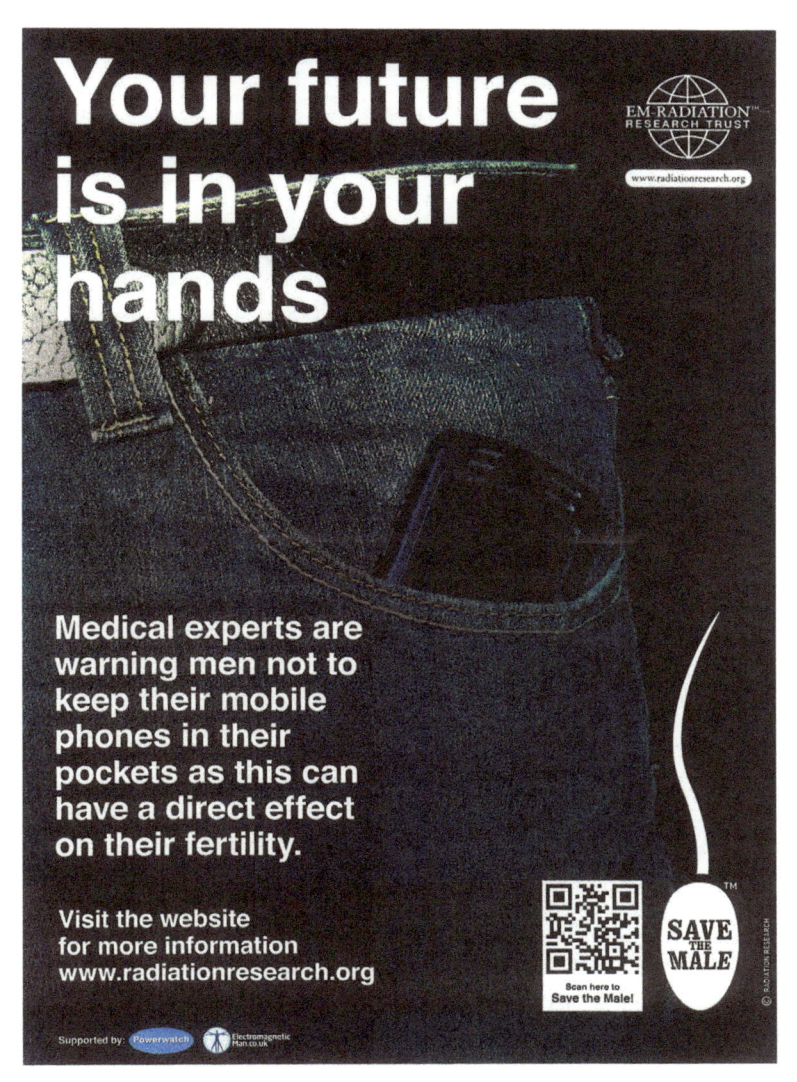

'Save the Male' – this RRT poster warning of the dangers to male fertility from mobiles in the pocket was deemed 'unacceptable' by the Advertising Standards Authority. *(Radiation Research Trust)*

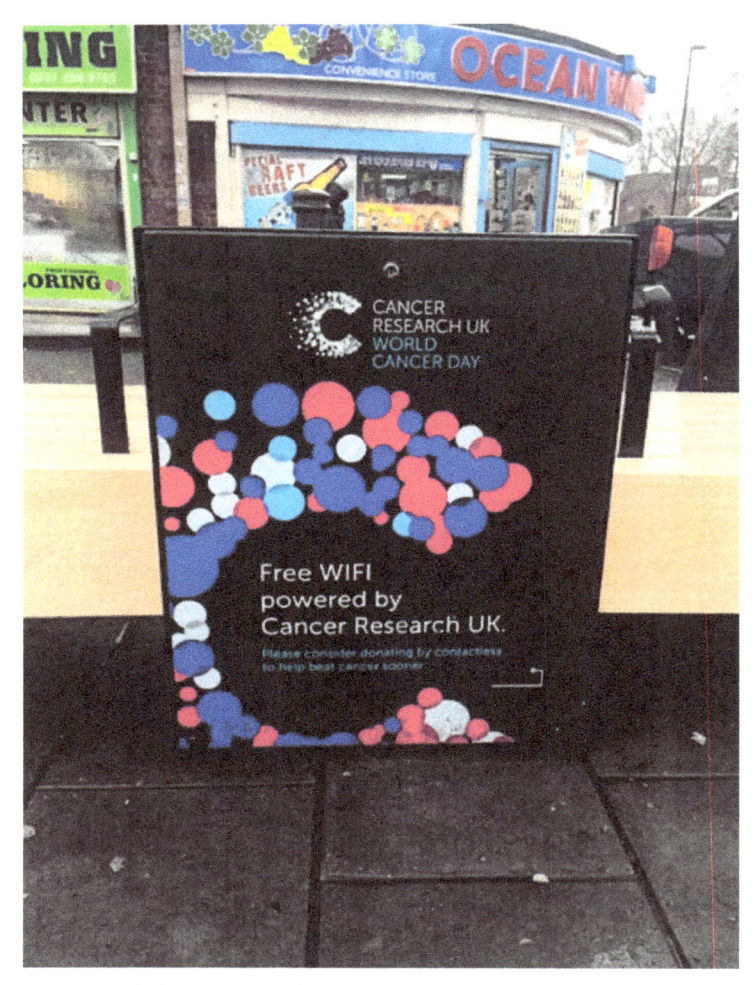

Cancer Research 'smart bench' poster in Islington, England. The charity has declared there is no link between cancer and wireless radiation. *(Radiation Research Trust/enhancement Damian Smith)*

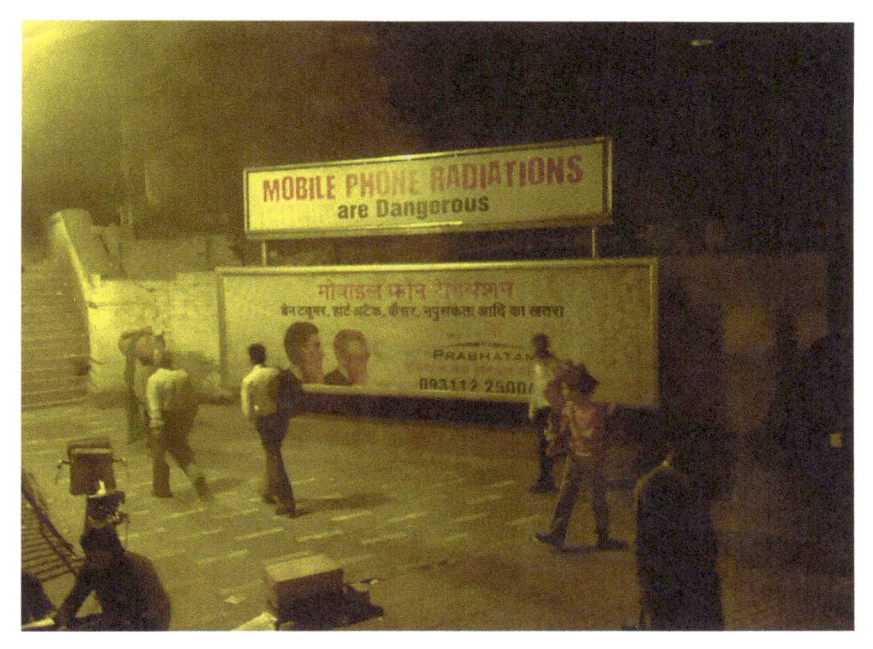

New Delhi railway station, India – campaigns for better disclosure about the health hazards of mobiles and masts have sprung up around the world.
(Radiation Research Trust/enhancement Damian Smith)

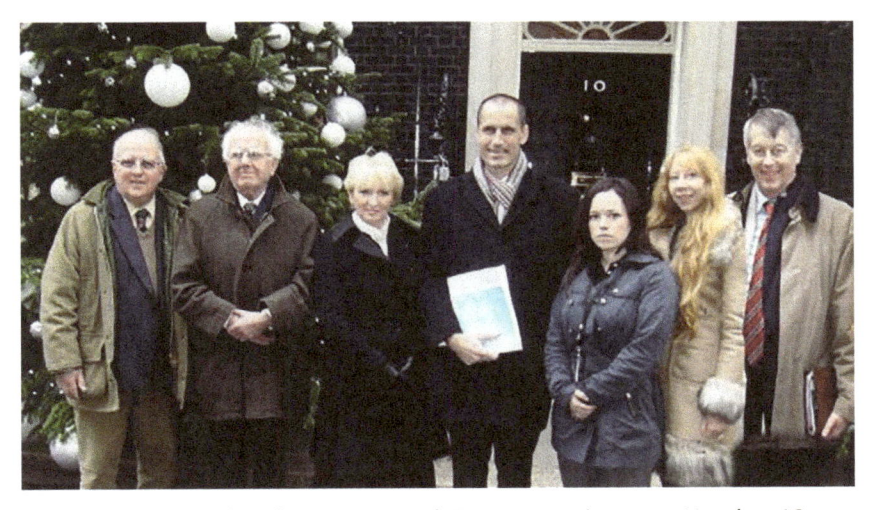

Brian Stein and Radiation Research Trust campaigners at Number 10 Downing Street. *(Radiation Research Trust)*

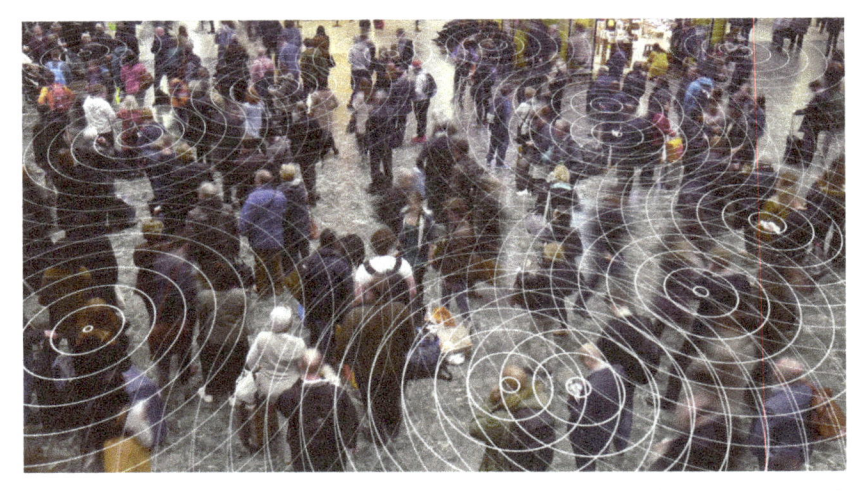

The range of microwave radiation from individual mobile phones in a typical public space. *(Peter Howell/Getty Images/istockphoto)*

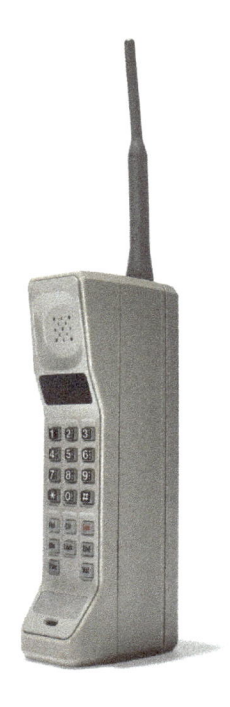

Early mobile phones were effectively untested for radiation safety levels and heavily marketed as prestige accessories. *(LiGo (uk))*

THE MICROWAVE DELUSION

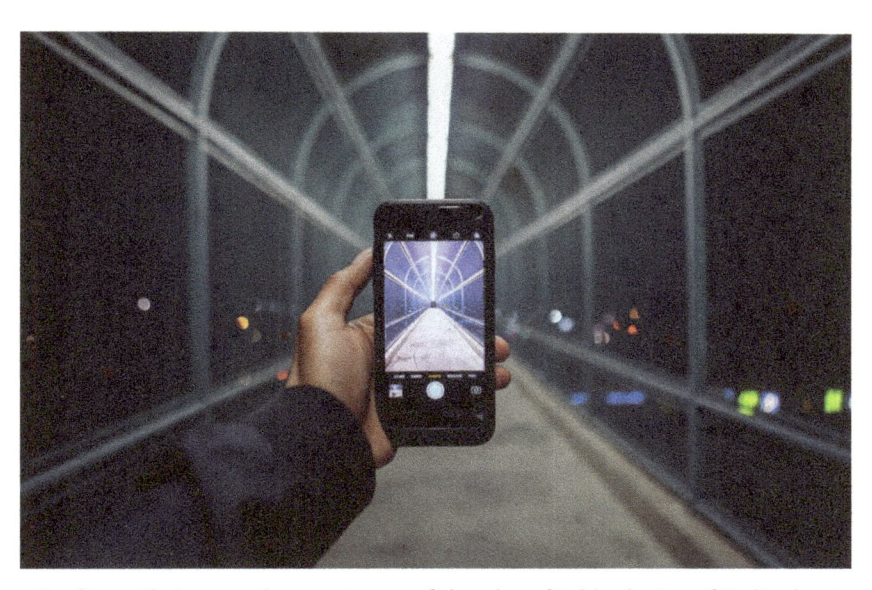

The 'Smart' phone – the most powerful and profitable device of its kind yet in mobile technology. *(Omar-Prestwich)*

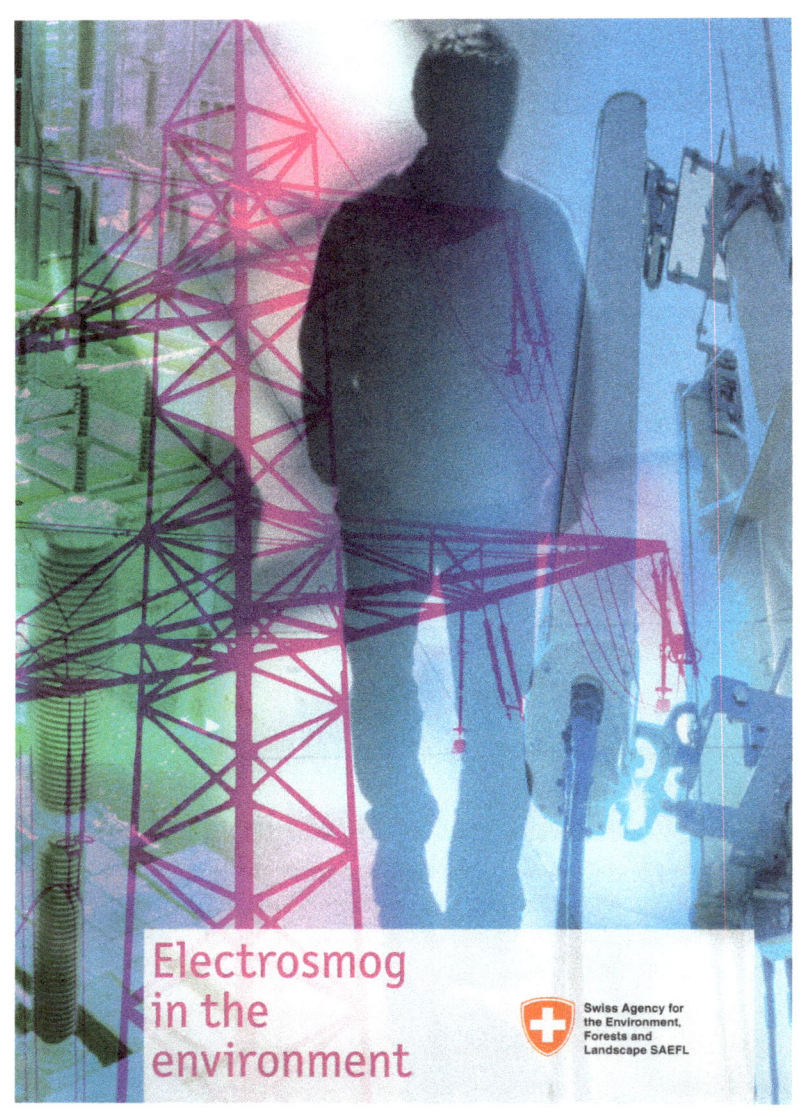

The Swiss government issued this booklet warning of the health hazards from wireless radiation to every citizen. *(Swiss Agency for the Environment, Forests and Landscape/picture conversion Damian Smith)*

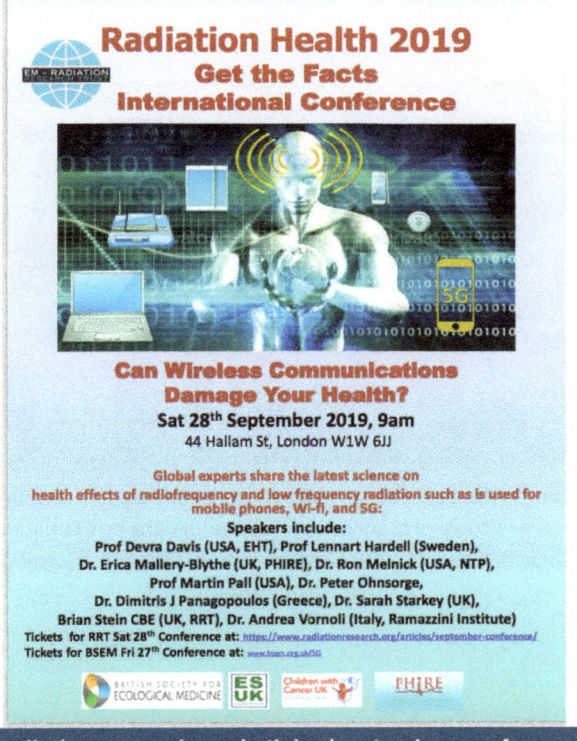

The 2019 Radiation Research Trust conference in London attracted delegates and leading independent scientists from all over the world. *(Radiation Research Trust)*

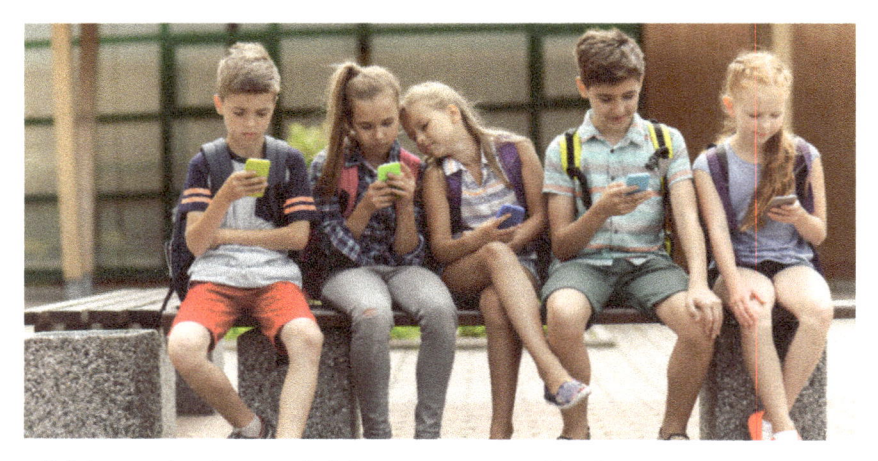

Children under the age of eighteen are targeted by the mobile industry and subject to peer group pressure: yet their skulls are not sufficiently formed to protect their brains from damage from non-thermal microwave radiation.
(Naturallysavvy.com)

4   Britons Enslav'd?

'I think the thing that shocked me the most was that up to that time, for about fifty years, I had thought the British government was on the side of the citizen – and therefore they would be looking after my interests. To discover that they knew what was going on, and they didn't warn me – there was no warning at all – I found more shocking than the thing itself.'

– Michael Bevington

'Unthinking respect for authority is the greatest enemy of truth.'

– Albert Einstein

Michael Bevington, Stowe School, England

Michael Bevington was head of Classics at Stowe School in Buckinghamshire, a leading co-educational boarding school set in a Palladian mansion with gardens by Capability Brown. Many 'Stoics' have gone on to become leading figures in the world of museums and the arts. Former pupils include Richard Branson – proprietor of among other things Virgin mobile.

Bevington was a neat, precise man with a sense of humour, who might have been expected to be bitter given the experiences that have befallen him. Nothing could have been further from the case. He was a popular head of department.

As chairman of ES-UK, he campaigned for ES people and greater transparency on the part of the British government with regard to the health effects of EMFs. Like Brian Stein, his principal weapons were experience, reason and a grasp of the facts, and his targets included the disregard for the same by those whom he believed owed citizens a duty of care.

He reserved his strongest criticism for the UK Health Protection Agency and British government scientists: 'They are the narrowest of the lot.'

'Being a teacher in my case is actually quite useful. I simplify things. And for this game you can't baffle people with science.'

'It was 2006. We have a group called the Rugby Group of schools which includes Stowe, Winchester etc. We meet every year and circulate every year. So I was away on the Thursday and on the Friday I came back here and they had put Wi-Fi into my classroom. It's an old orangery building with thick walls.'

'I came in on the Friday and thought, great, we can use it. I'd used it before once or twice and noticed that when one particularly large student walked in front of the machine in the corner everyone yelled at him: 'Oi, get out of the way! You're blocking the signal.'

'You never think about it – where the signal is going, what it is doing. I'd never thought, how can you sit in here and use a mobile phone? Where does the signal go? Through the wall? Through that window?'

'So by the end of that Friday in the newly-WiFi'd classroom I was getting headaches like I'd never had before,' (Bevington is a lean, fit hockey coach). 'We'd have Saturday morning lessons and it happened again. Then I came back on the Monday and it happened again and I thought, this is really weird.'

Bevington had the next lesson off, and someone had told him there was a meeting of the health and safety committee at lunchtime. He went online and searched 'Headaches and Wireless LAN'. Among his search results was the website of ES-UK.

'I thought, this isn't too good. The headaches built up over the course of that week. I remember lying awake in bed one night – I just couldn't sleep. It was so clearly the Wi-Fi – having found a case within three days on the internet. This chap had lost his job and he had exactly the same symptoms – this thudding headache, pains all round the body, heart palpitations... you just feel completely out of it.'

'I remember thinking, I can't go on with this. I spoke to my mother on the phone and she said, what's the point of teaching if you're in that state?'

'But I had three children - you don't want to give up your job. This seemed to be something else, it was completely new to you and you don't know any of its background whatsoever.'

Bevington decided to take advice from the medical profession: 'I think I saw about five doctors in the first few weeks. I went to the local practice – one doctor said: 'You fall between occupational and clinical.' They blamed the school and said it was their job to sort it out.'

'Another GP said: 'This is a political hot potato', but wouldn't elaborate. In a strange sort of way, I found this quite reassuring.'

Bevington also spoke to the school doctor, who was sympathetic and knew him to be no hypochondriac, but who seemed unwilling to countenance a physical explanation for his symptoms.

'Anyway, by the end of that week I decided I was going to do something.'

Bevington wrote a letter to the Headmaster 'saying I couldn't continue teaching with Wi-Fi. I thought, he's going to be in an awkward situation because he won't know what to do with it. So I put together a document to go with it.'

'He wouldn't see me immediately – he probably wanted to consult other people. He saw me at the end of the day and he said very decently – well he had to, duty of care as an employer – yes, we will remove it.'

'It then took at least a week because we hadn't realised how far this stuff had gone – through walls, other buildings. It later emerged that they had turned the Wi-Fi up to the maximum because they assumed quite correctly that we had these enormous thick walls. There was a base station in my room turned up to the maximum.'

'In a curious way, I am grateful that it was absolutely clear-cut.'

His symptoms did not abate: 'The body got more and more sensitive. I'd wake up at 3am in a complete state. I went to sleep at someone else's house. Then you begin to realise – we'd put in cordless phones and all that.'

'About a fortnight after that I had an hour before a hockey match and I rang ES-UK. As a bloke I am not inclined to discuss health. And they said: 'Look (a) you've got it for life and (b) your family's got it for life.' And they were absolutely correct.'

'I then realised that our neighbours had Wi-Fi, they had cordless phones. The houses were quite close together. The chap next to me had a home hub turned up quite high and it was going straight into our bedroom where our heads were.'

'I thought about moving house, but prices had gone up a lot.'

Bevington's Headmaster was in a difficult position: 'He could have turned round and said 'The Health Protection Agency says there's nothing wrong, leave.' But he had experienced unexpected health problems and he was sympathetic. His sister was a nurse. He had also been at Cambridge in the 80s, where a lot of people went straight into the City with the early mobile phones and ended up dead from brain tumours.'

'Quite a lot of the children at the school have parents who work in the mobile phone industry. We have a child whose father is the CEO of Sony. We have a grandchild of the Murdochs. The last thing they want is to upset the applecart.'

'So I told the Head I was going to speak out.'

Bevington's interview appeared in the *Times* on 26 November, 2006. This was the first time a wireless radiation story had appeared in the newspaper and it went all around the world:

'Yes, parents who read the *Times* might well worry about the welfare of their children. You're absolutely right. It's not my fault. It's their fault. I rang up the Health & Safety Executive as everyone does, asking them to sort it out, and we discover it's the UK Health Protection Agency and the Government blocking, right at the top. I suspect in the end it comes from America, like the Gulf War.'

'I understand David Cameron has been told by someone who spent half an hour with him in his surgery about the dangers of Wi-Fi, and he went home and said: 'Okay, I'm going to rip it out.'

By this time even Bevington, with some reason, was becoming a little paranoid: 'The story came out and things got quite interesting. I had some really good stuff thrust into my pocket while I was in a local restaurant. It was a photocopy of part of a document about the installation of Wi-Fi in schools. It was advocating Wi-Fi. At the end of the document, it said: *'A lot of our engineers doing this have gone down with headaches.'*

In spite of his misgivings about the freedom of the press, he sent the document to the *Times Educational Supplement*:

'It was the last day of term and they left a message on the school answerphone. I didn't get it and got home and my daughter Elizabeth was on the phone. She said: 'Dad, I can hardly hear this person! There are all these clicks on the phone!' Then it turned out that someone had been listening in on the school phone message as well.'

'It went through my mind, if I do something about this, I could be a target – it was a simple as that.'

'I think the thing that shocked me the most was that for about fifty years I had thought the government was basically on the side of the citizen – and therefore they would be looking after my interests. To discover that they knew what was going on and they didn't warn me – there was no warning at all – I found more shocking than the thing itself.'

'It didn't make sense. That is something I find incredibly difficult. No-one in the medical profession in this country, apart from a handful, is prepared to stand up.'

'I pressed the local surgery and they said, we will refer you to a consultant. They sent me to Stoke Mandeville. I went down with my wife, we had an hour, I explained all these things, how I hadn't known what was going on, then discovered it was Wi-Fi and mobile phones. At the end of it all he said: 'It's anxiety.'

'I don't think I've ever felt so shattered in my life. A professional person, who couldn't face the evidence, who hasn't got any guts.'

By this time Bevington had invested in a protective wire mesh at home. It looked odd, but it worked: 'I'd sleep under it and use it in the evening as well. As I went under it, I could feel the difference. I can't now – the sensitivity has accelerated.'

'How come I haven't gone nuts? A sense of humour. And also because eventually they are going to come such a cropper.'

'I have found in dealing with people the worst are the scientists by a long, long way. If you put forward some of the views that they do in the world of classics or history, they would be absolutely laughable. They are so blind, it is extraordinary. James Rubin at King's, for example, he's just *wrong*, full stop.'

'There hasn't been a Telecoms Act in this country since 1994. It's exactly what happened in the States. In France, they don't accept it and they can throw masts out purely on the grounds that people are worried about them.'

'Yes, we live in one of the most undemocratic countries in the world. It is amazing.'

Bevington remained appreciative of the school's enlightened stance: 'I have said to the school, whether you like it or not, you are one of the few schools that know about radiation effects and have actually acted on it.'

'They are desperate to have Wi-Fi in the boarding houses. And London insurers are already talking about what happens if Wi-Fi does turn out to be cancerous – and it already is – in ten years' time every parent will sue.'

So why didn't the mobile providers simply lower the SAR rates and change the technology?

'Absolutely, that's what I would do. I would say to the mobile people, every two years we will halve it, or whatever. We have the knowledge. These things can operate at incredibly low level.'

'One of the reasons Wi-Fi is so bad is that it pumps out at full power all the time.'

In Bevington's opinion, the threat to pupils was getting worse: 'In the evening, the children are sitting here and a lot of them are on their mobile phones. They are downloading stuff, talking to each other, to friends.'

'Back in March 2012 I felt a *ping* going through that doorway there – it's a bit like water I think, it flows wherever it can – I thought no more about it, and the next day I couldn't get out of bed. I felt nauseous and I was sick for the rest of the day – never known it before.'

'Then September, on duty again in here, all fine. Next day, spinning head, the works. I said to the school, I can't go on like this.'

'I discovered that around May they'd put in some new Wi-Fi routers. I had a measuring device and I was sitting in my classroom. *Ping, ping*, every now and again. Last term it was quite bad, this term it's baddish – I think it's all these new smartphones. They've got Wi-Fi, they've got Bluetooth, they talk to each other. They've got satnav and GPS.'

'So just imagine it. At the end of a lecture, everyone gets up with their phone on and moves. Up to 100 iphones – *ping, ping, ping* – all over the place. And I sit there in my study and I can't see these people, but the thing is shooting up to 0.8 volts per metre. That's actually way over the legal limit in some countries.'

'And no-one knows. No-one knows. People write to DEFRA – have you measured ipads? No, because they're safe, they're within the legal limits.'

'So I think actually there is going to be massive ill-health in the nation within however long it takes to work through, or it's going to change the genome, or whatever.'

'One good thing here, because we own all the land, the nearest masts are a long way away. They were doing some filming here. It was slightly drizzly and that changes all the electrics in the area. They had two or three hundred people here and they were between here and the hockey game where I was. It was about 3pm and we were three all and keen and suddenly three of them said 'I don't feel well, sir.'

'I'd already felt a *ping* and I thought, this is most odd, because there are no mobile phones anywhere around here. These three said they were ill, so I said, 'Okay, you can't go back to the house, you've got to sit here, on the damp grass, and it's three all.' And they said: 'Yes.'

'At the end I said, well what's wrong with you?

'We don't know, sir. We just feel odd, headache, all sorts of weird things.'

'Now what happened at 3.15pm down at the filming? Okay chaps, break. Just phoning home, everybody! 300 mobile phones switch on!

'My son, who is not sensitive, was running up by the arch over there. He had a nosebleed. It's on the way to where the mast is. And if you draw a line from my hockey match on the brow of the hill here, it's smack in the middle.'

'I think it will take David Cameron and co to go down with this illness until they actually take it seriously.'

'It's legal, and you can't under modern rules stop children communicating with home.'

'Sir William Stewart in 2000 said no child under 15 should use a mobile phone except in emergency. So we're trying to get Ofsted to take this up, but they won't, because they are being pushed around by the Department of Health.'

'The only thing that ever changes anything of this nature is money – that and the law courts. Mobile phones are unquestioningly allowed and masts are unilaterally imposed with a nice big cheque to the farmer or whoever.'

'So what does one do? I just continue. I teach Classics. I do my bit. You can't predict the future. The government will have to solve this one. And the longer they leave it, the bigger the hole they are digging.'

'The atmosphere's changed. The children were sceptical. They'd go around waving their phones at me, saying can you feel it? I gave a talk, with all these figures, and it meant absolutely nothing to them. Then I switched on my acoustimeter and said, just switch your phone on will you? *WHEEEEE!* What was that?'

'So they don't wave their phones at me any more.'

'They are now teaching this in schools in other countries, not here.'

'What is the role of government? Surely to protect the people. That includes wealth. But not actually to do them harm.'

'I think shareholders in mobile phone companies will dump their shares when they realise.'

'You go into teaching because you value people. I have Christian views, and I value truth. And I really do believe the truth will come out. It will eventually happen.'

'We are setting up a group now for teachers and lecturers at places like Oxford. They've all written to the UK Health Protection Agency: they're not interested. Their response is: 'Go to your doctor.'

5 Doctor, Doctor

'You need enough science to convince a GP'

– Dr Andrew Tresidder

Erica Mallery-Blythe: A Life in the Day, Lincolnshire, England

Erica Mallery-Blythe is a former Accident and Emergency doctor who lives with her RAF pilot husband and their daughter in Lincolnshire.

While she was living in America, Dr Mallery-Blythe worked with Dr Andrew Marino, one time research student of two-time Nobel nominee Dr Robert Becker, author of 'Crosscurrents' and 'The Body Electric'.

Dr Marino was also a key figure in the 1979 exposure of the irradiation of the US Embassy in Moscow. His work and reputation for rigour became a strong influence: 'Everybody has the potential to become electro-hypersensitive,' Dr Mallery-Blythe observes, 'Every cell in our body, in our brain, or nervous system is dependent on electrical signals. But some people have that extra sensitivity, and though they may not know it, it is causing their asthma, flu-like symptoms or insomnia.'

'Many people may be electro-hypersensitive and not realise it.'

The symptoms of electrohypersensitivity can be sporadic, making them difficult to track. So what can sufferers do if they believe the world is poisoning them?

'The only way to alleviate symptoms is to avoid the electromagnetic waves they feel cause them. Don't keep electronic devices in the room you sleep in, and switch off as many devices as you can in the house.'

'It is an appalling truth that people are being certified under the Mental Health Act because of their electrosensitivity. I know a 24 year-old stonemason to whom this happened. Among other things, as a result he was placed in a highly EMF environment. And being certified insane stays on your record. Yes, health service professionals are signing off these orders.'

Dr Mallery-Blythe, with health and education professionals and other concerned parties in the United States, Canada, France and South Korea, sees the greatest hazard from microwave radiation as being to the unborn child, young children and teenagers.

'There has been a huge escalation in children's symptoms such as autism with the rise in EMFs. EHS people are an advanced warning system of something that threatens all of us.'

'There are suicides, not surprisingly. The mother wrote to me of the boy (Michael Nield) who killed himself.'

'I have literally held life and death in my hands as I breathed air into new sets of tiny, silent lungs and in those moments we are prone to having the misconception that we understand the complexity of human life. In many crude senses we do and that is very useful, but there is so much to be learned.'

'The current physics framework regarding non-ionising radiation that we teach our doctors, scientists, engineers and children is simply wrong. We teach them that its power to harm biology is akin to its visibility... non-existent. We teach them that all good practice must be 'evidence-based', and yet, when the evidence is inconvenient, suddenly it is reasonable to disregard it entirely and instead be led by purses and politicians.'

'I am witnessing a grand betrayal of the science I was taught to respect so deeply. The evidence base for serious harm to health of humans, plants and animals from non-ionising radiation exposures is vast. Who are the responsible persons within WHO, ICNIRP, the Department of Health or Public Health England that are accountable for their 'mistakes'?'

'Early warning scientists and doctors are witch-hunted to silence, robbed of their research grants and labelled 'luddites' and scaremongers. In seducing the public to pay for this technological revolution it is sold as 'advancement', 'progress' and the inevitable 'future'... however if one adds the evidence base into these suggestions, 'advance in rate of neurodegenerative disease', 'progressively more sterility', a 'future rise in childhood cancers and neurodevelopmental disorders', it sounds a little less sexy.'

Dr Andrew Tresidder, Somerset, England

'When we all feel healthy, our vitality level is *up there* – when I was a junior doctor working 100 hours a week, mine suddenly went *down here*, and I felt absolutely knackered for three months. This was about twenty-five years ago. It was not like me at all.'

'The environment was unhealthy. I gradually rebuild my energies two or three years on and looked into complementary therapies. This went on for about five years, and none of these therapies are recognised by the Health Service.'

Dr Andrew Tresidder is a General Practitioner who combines conventional medicine with a disregard for its narrower orthodoxies. A warm man, a listener, good with people of all ages, he was the kind of GP most patients would want.

'I'd say the three big gaps in healthcare are, one, complementary therapies and health in general, two, is the pathology of the psyche, that is to say how it is possible to get out of balance or get stuck, and how it is possible to be rebalanced gently, and three, nutrition.'

'So, yes, I'm a GP and you come in and say I need some more pills doc, and I give them to you. Although I take a very empowering way with patients. I don't want you to come through the door and hand me the power.'

'So there are six questions for the patient. What is it? Why me? Why now? What's going to happen? What are you going to do?

And the sixth one, which I always add, is what can I (the patient) do?'

'If you hand back a bit of power you give back the locus of control. People don't come in wanting you to take the locus of control forever – if you have a chest infection, you need antibiotics. If you've got a broken leg, it needs fixing. You need good service, but you're not their client for ever.'

Over the years, he has developed a practice library of books on illness with a bias on how to help people help themselves. His general practice colleagues are tolerant, he says, because he 'cuts the mustard' on orthodox medicine.

Ten years ago, he went part-time from general practice and started to work in prisons. He also took a diploma in teaching medical education. He became a mental health-approved doctor and a patient safety lead for NHS Somerset. He also works with the police: 'and you have to be on the ball to do that.'

'So all this puts you within the system and being able to promote change.'

However, a few years ago, Dr Tresidder's personal system experienced change: 'You're a busy GP. You're stressed. I went away on holiday for two weeks, so your tension levels go right down. I came back, and the computer screens at work had been changed from black and white to colour. I sat about a foot away from them and I started feeling terrible. I thought, what's going on? I'd just had a holiday.'

'The same thing happened the next day. So I bought a flat screen monitor, which cost about £700, and I felt well again.'

Having acquired a mobile phone, he started to experience headaches and slurred speech. The same symptoms occurred when he used Bluetooth in the car: 'So I stopped using the mobile and it got better. No, I didn't think, oh God, have I had a stroke, do I have a brain tumour? I could recognise exactly the stimulus.'

Dr Tresidder recognised the colour screens and the mobile phone as triggers for his symptoms, but he did not know the symptoms' name. Then he came across the Powerwatch Handbook.

'So I learned about electrosensitivity. A lot of my knowledge has been driven by my personal circumstances. I mentioned the possibility about ten years ago to a director of nursing, and they said, 'Oh, yes, you're electrically sensitive.'

Dr Tresidder continued to use a flat screen hard-wired computer in his office at home. He also continued to use a mobile phone, albeit sparingly: 'I've diagnosed a few patients along these lines. I've helped people waking up with headaches get rid of them by moving the mobile out of the bedroom. It can be the television, it can be the DECT phone, it can be the computer.'

Dr Tresidder has largely succeeded in healing his own system and those of others. In terms of working within the wider system and promoting change, however, he is less optimistic.

'The NHS has gone from Beveridge and a generation of patients who had no experience or expectations of having things done for them, to a healthcare system dominated by the pharmaceutical companies. Government now has all these so-called 'advisors' – from the drug companies.'

'The pharmaceutical companies, although they don't like to admit it, actually spend more on marketing than they do on research.'

'I don't see drug company reps any more. They were often very attractive women with a hint of knee, and I'm a bloke. I used to interrupt their eye contact trick with the reply: 'I'm sorry, but I've heard that anyone who sustains eye contact for more than ten seconds is either about to attack you, or has designs on your body.'

In his opinion, too many GPs become entrenched in their positions: 'Man trained to use a hammer sees everything as a nail.' If you are trained in pharmacology, you don't think about geopathic stress as a cause. ES is all about 'not invented here' syndrome when it comes to the NHS.'

'Governments first say there's no problem, then there's a problem but it's a very small problem, then there is a problem, and then, oh my God, there's a problem. Then it's time for another government.'

'When was there last a decent Health Secretary? I think it was in about 1967 – but he was the son of a doctor.'

'The car was not invented to be safe, it was invented to sell. Lots of people died. Only consumer pressure eventually forced car manufacturers to introduce seat belts. It's the same with mobile phones.'

'Scientists go where the money is. If the money says, prove it doesn't exist, they'll prove it. If I said to someone, can I put up a mast in your back garden? They would reply in two words, the second of which would be 'off'. But if I say, can I put in a home hub, with multiple Wi-Fi etc, all for £12.50 a month, they would reply, 'Yes, please!'

As to the question of ES and its effects: 'Why does music affect us in the way it does? We don't know – but we know it does.'

'Society has abrogated responsibility for health. Individually and collectively, we are playing out a Faustian tragedy. We have a fourfold responsibility – to ourselves, our colleagues, our immediate environment and the wider environment. In this sense, there's never been a better time to develop yourself.'

'Are future generations going to live longer? The answer is no. They are going to age faster. In terms of the effects of electromagnetic fields on DNA, five or six years down the road we are looking at wide-scale catastrophe.'

'Yes, I was a conventional GP. I got less conventional as time went on'. Dr. Diana Samways, Haslemere, Surrey, England

Dr Samways is a brisk, cut-glass-voiced, bridge-playing, oratorio-singing sixty-something of the sort you would want as an aunt or a godmother. She had attended the 2011 ES-UK conference in Melton Mowbray and been shocked at what she witnessed. Like Dr Mallery-Blythe, she is strongly critical of the forced incarceration of electrically sensitive people by the NHS in mental hospitals, and clinical environments containing high levels of electromagnetic fields.

In the 1980s, Dr Samways was a General Practitioner in Haslemere: 'Yes, I was a conventional GP. I got less conventional as time went on.'

She worked for the NHS, and began to develop a private practice. She also trained in drink and drug rehabilitation in the United States. Back in Haslemere, she began to experience night terrors and panic attacks: 'It sort of crept up. Nobody seemed to know about it. Eventually I realised there was something wrong with this house. I was allergic to mould.'

'I think you are often sent what you are meant to deal with. So I was dealing with mould allergy and irritable bowel syndrome, which I think are connected.'

These areas became Dr Samways' professional constituency, practicing from her house – which she had treated for mould – and in the process gaining insights into the therapeutic shortcomings of pharmaceutical company-driven standard medicine. She also became a screening doctor for BUPA, the private healthcare provider: 'In my home practice I was dealing with alcoholism and drug addiction, and all the anorexics started to come. This was by word of mouth. Yes, I had a desire to treat people who to some degree were not getting properly treated by the NHS.'

Then electrosensitivity, as she put it, 'came onto my radar.'

'So ES people started to come. A woman who wore a beehive hat called me on the phone and I said, 'I can probably help you.'

'What I try to do for ES people is reduce the total load on the body. I mean by this all the things we do, the stuff we eat, we breathe, the mobile phonery, all that is total load. You get a donkey cart carrying everything including the kitchen sink: the donkey falls to its knees. You take some of the load off, the donkey gets up again.'

'People need to tell me quite a lot about their lifestyles. I see them for an hour, I listen and they usually tell me the answer. They usually know. I can add things occasionally. They shake my hand and look me in the eye and say, 'You are the first doctor who has ever listened to me.'

'I can help ES people by telling them what they can turn off and what they can do about the house, the car. A taxi driver from London came to see me. He had every conceivable gadget in his cab: he couldn't work with it and he couldn't work without it.'

'Friends call me up, and say they think there is a problem with their house. They have Wi-Fi and they have DECT phones. All these things are measurable. Before 2001 they were analogue phones: you can still buy reconditioned ones from a place in Devon. Or off eBay.'

'So I go in there with my bit of kit and measure and say, if you took that out... and we pull it out and there is a difference. For measuring microwaves, I use an acoustimeter. The first thing I do is get people onto Site Finder, which tells you where the mobile phone masts are.'

'One of the people I visit has a Tetra mast right outside her home and she's been diagnosed with MS – she's youngish.'

Dr Samways is critical of the relationship between local authorities and mobile providers: 'They just put up these masts. They haven't updated Site Finder since 2006. Why is that? And why, if they are so safe, are they disguising masts as green boxes in the street?'

She is equally sceptical of the safety claims of consumer technology: 'Don't put it in your lap. It shouldn't be called a laptop.'

'It is a shocking truth that people suffering from electrosensitivity are being certified by the NHS. I have had phone calls in the middle of the night from mental hospitals from people wanting to know how they can get out. Yes, they have severe problems, but they are not manic depressives: they are suffering as a result of electrosensitivity. In each case, health service professionals have signed off these orders.'

In reply to the common industry defence, she says: 'The first few cases of bubonic plague were 'anecdotal.'

Dr Samways has published widely. She continues her electrosensitivity consultations in the community. The ageing demographics of Surrey, however, are against her: 'Most people I see are over fifty, so they don't have young children at home. I show them the source of the problem and in many cases they don't take the slightest notice. The technology is too convenient. I think it will just have to get worse in order for people to realise.'

'The Body is a Halfwave Dipole': The Undercover Epidemiologist, London, England

'You have to think about how electrosensitivity predates the wireless and even the electrical age – the symptoms go back centuries - ancient sites of electrosensitive behaviour, interpreted as mysterious afflictions and assuming folkloric status. Dorset, Somerset; depressions, suicides; animals becoming dysfunctional. It's geophysical, mineral. The *genius loci*.'

'We are all accidental antennae. The body is a halfwave dipole.'

The Undercover Epidemiologist and a colleague carry out measurements around Tetra and multiplex masts across the country. Their work is conducted covertly: if this was 1941, they would probably have been in Occupied Europe working for SOE.

'We stop the car, and when somebody comes out and asks us what we are doing, we say, 'We hear you've been having trouble with your television reception and we've been subcontracted to investigate.' 'Oh, yes!' They say. And we find microwave radiation levels way above what they should be.'

'As we get to know one another better, you'll know more about what I mean when I say I have sent things 'up the line'.

'There's a formula for measuring the beam from multiplex and Tetra masts. Once you know the height, you can work out the angle of the beam and exactly where it hits the ground and you can go there to take the measurement.'

'I've been on one of the UK Health Protection Agency committees for years. The electromagnetic field discussion group - I still feed into that.'

'Yes, the amounts of money involved on both sides and in the middle – George Carlo for example - confuse the picture. You know about the Interphone Study: about how the Danish study excluded the businessmen users. COSMOS and the Essex Trials: again the methodology was seriously flawed.'

'Yes, Italy is the most unlikely country to have dropped the safety levels to a better place, enabling Marcolini to win his case.'

'I keep my field operative stuff very low profile. It goes up the line. I do a lot of work on brain tumours.'

There is much talk of sine waves and the flawed methodological approach of British government researchers: 'Why? I think it's lack of knowledge, lack of rigour. In the case of Essex, the room was newly decorated so there was effect from the paint. They'd done the walls, but not the floor. So it wasn't a true Faraday chamber.'

'The mentality of 'we know better'? Where does that come from? I think they are interested in protecting our own fiefdoms.'

In Germany, the UE investigated a childhood leukaemia cluster in a hamlet on the bank of the River Elbe. There was a nuclear power station on the other side.

'But it wasn't the power station that caused it - it was the radar and microwave masts on the ships going up and down the Elbe - because of the level of the river, they were exactly at the level of the hamlet.'

'The Germans are very much ahead of the UK on masts and cancer clusters.'

The Undercover Epidemiologist has investigated radio hams and breast cancer clusters; cancer clusters among farmers who have been paid to have masts sited on their land. He/she worries worries about toxins and stress; about how valuable trace elements such as selenium and zinc have been ploughed out of the soil – 'We should take supplements' – about the effects of the new edimium magnets in i-players on young users.

'Remedies to electrosensitivity in the home can be applied successfully – yes!'

The Undercover Epidemiologist has a high security clearance. We have to assume he/she is speaking with authority.

'The truth is, there is no precedent for this as a public health matter. And believe me, this is a matter of public health.'

6 The Scientific Silence (Why Microwaves Cause Cancer in Russia, China, India and Italy, and Are 'Safe' in Britain)

'The absence of evidence is not evidence of absence.'

– Carl Sagan

In Europe, Italy, Luxembourg, Switzerland, Austria and parts of Belgium had all tightened the acceptable safety thresholds. With China and India, soon half the world's population would have done the same.

Why not Britain?

Britain is situated at the crossroads of independent scientific traffic – in the east from Professor Yuri Grigoriev in Russia, Professor Lennart Hardell and Professor Olle Johansson in Sweden and Professor Dariusz Leszcynski in Finland; in the west from Professor Joel Moskowitz, Cindy Sage in California, Dr Martha Herbert at Harvard and Dr Magda Havas in Canada. But Britain seems not have their equivalents. Or, if it does, the voices are silent.

Brian Stein: 'There's a connection – I don't know quite what it is – between Essex University and Kings College London. A number of people there will regularly spout on about ME, Gulf War syndrome, and say they're all psychological. They do the tests to prove that. It's almost as if they're guns for hire.'

'Yes, the funding comes from the government, and at the end of the day it might otherwise lay them open to massive legal claims – correct.'

'Why is there a difference here between say Sweden and the UK? We are both democracies. Alasdair Philips would say it is because of our nuclear heritage and the military vested interest. The UK Health Protection Agency was born out of the radiation research which was born out of the nuclear age and the Cold War. So okay, we've moved on, but the culture is still the same. And Sweden has never been a nuclear power.'

'Also, we defeated the IRA with mobile phone technology. The mobile phone industry must have been hand in glove with the government.'

'And that's fine, to defend our country. But we're now rolling it (the peril) out twice over.'

'I think the countries that are the most anti the truth are the ones that are most dependent on the military. So America and the UK can't allow people to think that we're damaging our soldiers. Whereas Switzerland… does it have an army? Likewise, where are all the major telephone companies? In America and the UK – not Switzerland. For them it's not such a problem, telling the truth.'

In Britain, the UK Health Protection Agency and mobile providers had persuaded the media and the public that the 'psychological' approach to electrosensitivity and electrohypersensitivity was the appropriate one: thus the work of Dr James Rubin at Kings College London, Elaine Fox and the Essex Trials, Professors Challis, Coggan *et al.*

Professor Challis, chairman of the Mobile Telecommunications and Health Research Programme (MTHRP), funded by the British Government and the mobile phone industry, had managed to convince himself and the media that he was 'independent of both.' Yet, as we have seen, his so-called 'independent' findings were directly at odds with those of genuinely independent researchers.

Of the MTHRP's five year research into the 'short-term' effects of mobile phones and masts, Challis had declared: 'These are high quality studies, and the signs are that they do not show any short-term effects from exposure to mobile phones.'

As Brian Stein had discovered, there was one 'truth' for electrically sensitive people and another for government and industry-backed scientists and researchers.

'When extra sensitive people' (Challis seemed to acknowledge that they existed) 'are placed in conditions where they do not know whether a mobile phone is on or off, they are unable to tell more often than you would expect.'

Brian Stein would question this.

'This needs further investigation,' Challis conceded, 'Cancer takes more than ten years to appear: we have seen that with cigarettes, asbestos and the atomic bomb... We have no evidence so far of harm coming from mobile phones, but that does not mean that there is no harm... Short-term experiments do not tell us much about long-term effects. The only sure way of finding out whether there are long-term effects is to study people's health over a long period.'

Yet in Britain's academic institutions, which had produced so many great scientists and Nobel Prizewinners, the conditions under which these long-term effects could be scientifically tested either no longer existed, or were created not by independent scientists but by psychologists with a different agenda.

Like Professor Challis, Dr Rubin at Kings College London was funded by the mobile phone industry through the MTHR research programme, which effectively channelled industry money to scientists such as Professor Challis and researchers such as Dr Rubin so that they could seem to be 'independent'. Flawed or discredited studies such as Interphone and Cosmos had also been funded in this way.

Professor Andrew Goldsworthy (**See link in Appendix 2**) was a retired lecturer from Imperial College, London, renowned for its expertise in electrical engineering and health. He had spent years studying calcium metabolism in living cells and also how cells, tissues and organisms are affected by electrical and electromagnetic fields.

Professor Goldsworthy had published widely in peer-reviewed journals and supervised many undergraduate and Ph.D students. But when (later Dr.) Heather Whitney, a third-year undergraduate, co-authored a paper with Professor Goldsworthy on the biological effects of conditioned water, which led to his explanation of the mechanism of the biological effects of mobile phones, there was an abrupt reaction. As Professor Goldsworthy recalled: 'I subsequently published it with her as a co-author, and it was considered to be so important by the mobile phone industry that I was not allowed to have any more research students and my laboratory facilities at Imperial College were to all intents and purposes closed down.'

Professor Goldsworthy's experience recalled that of Allan Frey and Om P. Gandhi in the United States in the 1970s and 1980s. America had moved on since then; Britain had not.

The independent science in Britain by the likes of Professor Goldsworthy, Professor Denis Henshaw and others confirming the harmful physiological effects of radio frequency radiation, largely mirrored the findings of non-industry scientists and healthcare professionals in the United States, Canada, Sweden, Finland, Russia, France and Belgium. Yet the British research had all but been closed down. Why should this be so?

Another explanation may lie in the fact that countries such as America, Canada, Sweden and Denmark had strong public sector economies and unions in areas of teaching and public health – with concomitantly strong lobbying powers and freedom of information. In Britain, the effective privatisation of these areas over the last three decades had had many benefits, but left regulatory powers and the raising of awkward questions in the hands of the free market and powerful private sector interests.

Combined with traditions – possibly delusions - of secrecy and self-importance hung over from the Cold War and Northern Ireland, these were powerful obstacles to independent long-term research into radio frequency radiation. As Alasdair Philips of Powerwatch noted as far back as 2011:

'The industries which are major users of spectrum are themselves significant contributors to the economy. Key sectors of the wireless industry generated **revenue totalling £37.3 billion** in 2011 and contributed **117,500 jobs**. In addition, mobile communications and other wireless applications are a significant component of the internet economy, which is growing rapidly, providing exciting opportunities for innovation and growth.'

'As an illustration, a recent study by AT Kearney found that the UK internet economy is worth £82 billion a year, equivalent to 5.7% of the country's gross domestic product. Mobile internet connections are growing in significance, accounting for 16% of the internet economy. Analysys Mason estimates that mobile data traffic in the UK has grown by 25% in the last year and that similar rates of growth will be maintained for the next five years. Other commentators, for example Cisco, are forecasting even more rapid growth in data traffic.'

'In the UK, the public mobile communications sector supports a supply chain of infrastructure, equipment, applications and content providers, generating annual revenue of around GBP20 billion (EUR24 billion) and supporting 75,000 jobs, while the broadcasting services sector supports a supply chain worth around GBP16 billion (EUR19 billion) per year and supports 40,000 jobs.'

By 2018, the value to the UK economy had risen to hundreds of billions, and the numbers of jobs had risen commensurately: albeit jobs in traditional sectors were being wiped out in the process.

Professor Goldsworthy agreed:

'It seems that our respective governments (perhaps because wireless telecommunications are seen as a cash cow and the Industry is too big to fail) are hell bent on either denying that any of these conditions exist or, if they do, they have nothing to do with electromagnetic exposure. This is why I made a point of saying that the annual cost of autism to the UK economy exceeds the annual tax revenue from the cell phone industry so, if the bulk *of ASD is due to microwave communications, the Government could close the whole industry down and still show a profit.'*

'There may be ways to mitigate some of the adverse effects of microwave telecommunications, but there is no guarantee that they will work in all cases and from what contacts I have had with the industry, they certainly do not want to try them out since it would presumably mean that these conditions actually exist and this could invite all sorts of litigation.'

With the colossal revenues to be had from the spread of wireless technology and corresponding gains to the Exchequer, this situation had suited mobile operators and successive governments, both of whom, for differing if obvious reasons, found it convenient to back the 'psychological' approach - and allegedly bad science – sponsored by the UK Health Protection Agency – which was itself dissolved in 2013 and replaced by Public Health England.

The consequence was that, in the context of the health hazards of wireless technology and radio frequency radiation, the government that was supposed to look after you, as expressed by Michael Bevington, Phil Inkley and others, was not there.

Brian Stein: 'If you just take on the industry-funded scientists, you're going to lose. They deliberately create confusion. If they can keep rebutting what somebody else says, the ordinary punter in the street remains confused. They love their mobile phones anyway and they want to believe the authorities that it's safe. That's what they want to believe. That's what I wanted to believe.'

'Where I get to now, having listened to one or two industry-funded scientists, I don't think that any piece of research that could be done showing how dangerous mobile phones are, would make ICNIRP or the UK Health Protection Authority or Public Health England go: 'Oh! They're might be a problem here.' They're not going to do that, no matter what. They're there to protect the economy.'

'What ICNIRP have done is a little bit like setting the road speed limit outside a primary school at one thousand miles an hour.

Then they can say, everyone's within the speed limit. People are being killed, but it's okay, they're within the limit.'

'So when the Italians lower the limit, as in the Marcolini case, the industry suddenly gets into problems.'

'Let's say for the sake of argument it's 'pyschological' or psychosomatic. My argument is this. If this had been psychosomatic, it would have become so with the emergence of electricity. People were frightened of electricity. It gave them an electric shock – but it didn't make them ES. 'Psychosomatic' people would have started saying, 'I'm allergic to electricity'. It didn't happen - until wireless came along – that's when people started being damaged.'

'There's no logic now in saying electrosensitive people suffer from a psychosomatic disorder' – had they been, they would have been so years ago, when they put up power lines.'

'In Britain, it is not 'politically correct' to listen for a number of reasons. One, I think the government thinks this problem is a very small one. Two, we're coming out of a recession. We don't want to know if there's a problem. Three, we sell off the next bandwidth spectrum and raise another £10 billion. And four, there's all this 'research' that keeps coming from the mobile phone industry that says everything's okay.'

'So it must be okay. We're all okay, aren't we?'

'And we're all okay, until we're not.'

In Russia, by contrast, a country that inspired fear and fascination in equal measure, with a history of repression, one-party rule and a reputation for expansionism and gangsterism, it would seem things were done differently.

7 Free Russia (Why the Former Communist World Leads the Way)

'Why is Russia able to accept that EMFs cause cancer while in the west it is impossible?'

'Russia has a long scientific tradition in this field - their researchers were national heroes and honoured scientists. In the UK and USA, any scientist who shows that EMFs cause cancer is ridiculed and denounced as a poor scientist, a campaigner, or has some vested interest.'

'In a communist state people do not generally have the right to go on strike, or sue for compensation from the state: so the fact that EMFs cause cancer is not economically damaging.'

'In the 'free' west, recognition that EMFs cause cancer would cause protests, danger money for workers in certain industries and litigation followed by significant economic damage.'

'When challenging the chief executive of 'Sense about Science' that EMFs cause cancer, I was told by her that if that was true we would have to 're-write the laws of physics!'

'Russia has accepted that EMFs cause cancer and has not had to re-write the laws of physics. What is it in the western psyche that has brainwashed us to believe that the only damage that can be caused by non-ionising radiation is by the heating effect?'

'This is the essence of the microwave delusion:'

'Free radicals damage DNA.'

'Non–ionising radiation can create free radicals.'

'Non-ionising radiation can therefore damage DNA.'

'Damaged DNA can cause cancer.'

'What has Russia to gain from admitting that EMFs cause cancer?'

'What has Britain and America to gain from denying that EMFs cause cancer - other than trillions of pounds and dollars?'

– Brian Stein

The notion that Russia protected its citizens against non-thermal microwave radiation better than the governments of America, Canada and Britain sounded unlikely, yet it was true. Russia's radio frequency radiation acceptable safety thresholds – like those of India, China, Italy, Switzerland, Bulgaria and other East European countries – were far lower than those of America, Canada and Britain.

Russian scientists had begun researching the biological effects of non-thermal radiation as far back as 1933 in response to symptoms of ill-health manifested in thousands of workers employed on military bases and in industrial plants. In this field, as in others, the then Soviet Union was technologically ahead of America.

Even when the Soviets irradiated the US Embassy in Moscow six to eight hours a day, five days a week from 1953 to 1976, resulting in unusually high incidences of cancers among Embassy staff, they had done so at a level – 18 microwatts - that was nearly double their own safety standard of 10 microwatts, but five hundred times lower than that which the US Department of Defense insisted was harmless.

Soviet research had continued through six decades and the country's metamorphosis into the Russian Federation. N. Rubtsova was a scientist at the RAMS Institute of Occupational Health in Moscow: his *Overview of Health Effects of Extremely Low Frequency Magnetic Fields* published in English revealed dozens of clinical and psychological studies carried out since the 1960s into the relationships between EMFs and a range of ailments in children and adults. The findings suggested links but were inconclusive and called for more research.

In 2000, the international workshop 'Clinical and physiological investigations of people highly exposed to electromagnetic fields' held in St Petersburg included the presentation by Valentina Nikitina of the North-West Scientific Centre of Hygiene and Public Health entitled 'Hygienic, clinical and epidemiological analysis of disturbances induced by radio frequency EMF in the human body'.

The conclusions are quoted in full:

'1. Performed studies suggest the identity of health disturbances among the workers exposed to low intensity HF and SHF EMR.'

'2. The disease induced by electromagnetic radiation is clinically manifested in vegetative dystonia syndrome with typical subjective complaints, disturbances in the central nervous system, cardiovascular system, reproductive system and gastrointestinal tract and biochemical changes in blood.'

'3 Revealed changes are persistent in character and do not disappear after ceasing the EMF exposure.'

'4. Early ageing syndrome observed in the group of HF-device regulators should be attributed to the remote effect of chronic RF EMF exposure. Polypathology, early development of age pathology, lipid metabolism disturbance, hormonal gonade function decrease, the character of thyol disulphide changes are the symptoms of ageing syndrome.'

'5. Hygienic assessment of exposure conditions and of accompanying workplace factors, consideration of social and living conditions, and dynamic health status follow-up are of utmost importance for the diagnosis of chronic EMR effects.'

The Russian National Committee on Non-Ionizing Radiation Protection had provided the first detailed summary in English of the most significant Russian research into radio frequency radiation and electromagnetic fields over the previous fifty years. According to the RNCNIRP, hazards likely to be faced by children who used mobile phones in the near future included disruption of memory, decline of attention, diminished learning and cognitive abilities, increased irritability, sleeplessness, increased sensitivity to stress and greater susceptibility to epilepsy.

The Deputy Chairman of RNCNIRP was Professor Oleg Grigoriev, Head of Department of Non-Ionizing Radiation, Director of the Federal Medical Biophysical Centre of the Federal Medical Biological Agency of Russia and Director of the Centre for Electromagnetic Safety:

'We need correct control and assessment of electromagnetic pollution,' he stated, 'There are currently a lot of new frequencies containing modulation and no one knows the results which could be a serious problem.'

Russian scientists were not only warning their own citizens, but ministries of health and other organisations around the world of the hazards of radiofrequency radiation, recommending hard-wired networks in schools and educational institutions instead of networks using wireless broadband systems.

In the Russian collective opinion, the ICNIRP guidelines were wrongly confined to short-term, acute thermal radiofrequency radiation and electromagnetic fields exposure. Both the ICNIRP and IEEE standards, in the Russian view, were based on the misleading and outdated position of governments and authorities such as those in America and Britain, that the only possible and established biological effect of RF/EMF exposure was tissue heating. Russian standards, by contrast, were supported by extensive research into non-thermal exposure and were backed by the Russian Ministry of Health: they were set at a fraction of the levels declared safe by ICNIRP and the IEEE which prevailed in America, Britain and many other countries.

Professor Grigoriev: 'We need to include non-Government groups in discussion and research. Non- Government groups play an equal importance to Government and the scientific community. NGOs are a new power and are representing people with electrosensitivity and should be an equal player.'

'If the decisions are not made together with the NGOs, then decisions may have no value.'

Pre-eminent in Russian thinking was the Chairman of the Russian National Committee on Non-Ionizing Radiation Protection and member of the World Health Organisation's International Advisory Committee on EMF and Health, Professor Yury Grigoriev. A living history of Soviet and Russian science, Professor Grigoriev delivered a message which for the first time was translated into English: 'Man conquered the Black Plague,' he declared, 'but he has created new problems - EMF pollution.'

Professor Grigoriev postulated *'Four indisputable truths to the risk assessment of mobile communications for public health.'*

'We have entered into active discussion for more than fifteen years about whether or not there are adverse effects as a result of exposures to mobile communications. Despite the discussions there is not progress, in my opinion.'

'However EMF exposures on the population are continuing, and a radiation loading grows daily.'

'Today I have chosen four postulates, or axioms, or absolute truths. These four truths are connected to mobile communications and, in my opinion, are essential for the population to fully understand the risk.'

'The first postulate *- mobile communications use EMF and RF. This kind of electromagnetic radiation is harmful and EMFs in all countries are stocked with appropriate regulations. Excess of allowable levels can cause pathology. I believe that you should agree that EMFs require restrictions and hygiene control!'*

'The second postulate *- "EMF and a brain". A mobile phone is an open EMF source without a protective shield. EMF is directly exposing the brain when we use a mobile phone. The nervous system structures of the internal ear (acoustical and vestibular devices) are directly exposed to the EMF beam.'*

'This kind of exposure of the brain has arisen for the first time in the history of civilization.'

'The third absolute truth *- "EMF RF and children".*

'Children, for the first time in civilization, are EMF-exposing their own brains.'

'The risk for damage to a child's brain compared to the adult brain is much greater.'

'Children are more vulnerable to external factors of the environment.'

'This is also the opinion of WHO (Backgrounder No3, 2003) and the Parma Declaration 2010 of the European Region of WHO.'

The fourth postulate is "Absence of adequate recommendation/standards".

'We have very little scientific material about the probable pathological effects after long-term EMF exposure on the brain of adults and children, so we have no scientific base for the definition of a permissable level of exposure on the brain to EMFs from mobile phones - and, as consequence, the corresponding standards are not there.'

'What is the solution?'

'For my suggestions, I have drawn on my experience and life time knowledge.'

'I have wide experience of research on issues surrounding two problems - " Ionizing radiation and health" (more than 60 years) and «Non-Ionizing radiations and health" (about 40 years).'

'I encountered the first issue in 1949. There were periods of 'underestimation, 'hyper assessment with elements of phobias, and again a period of 'underestimation' before the Chernobyl nuclear accident. This accident caused fear among the population. The Russian government agreed to provide full information to the population about the dangers of ionizing radiation. As a result the population of Russia is now reassured and respect decisions regarding protective actions.'

'Now we are dealing with similar issues surrounding EMF mobile communications. I believe that the time has arrived to provide full information to the general population.'

'These four postulates allow the population to appreciate the probable risk of adverse health effects from the uncontrolled use of mobile communications. Of course, we must remind people that their entire body is also continuously exposed round-the-clock to extra exposures associated with EMF base stations and Wi-Fi.'

'I think that mobile communications should be used only on a selective basis. Because of the dangers inherent in microwave technology, and the failure of standards to protect the population in general and particularly children, there should be the option of short term, temporary use so that we may preserve human health.'

'I say to my colleagues: do not sin against the truth. Deeds, not words!'

One Russian consumer who echoed these sentiments was Nikolai Lesnikov, a resident of the Moscow region, who took the Russian mobile operator MTS to court for installing a microwave tower twenty metres from his home. Lesnikov argued the company had 'abused his constitutional right to a favourable environment' and demanded that the tower be taken down.

MTS argued that the radiation from base stations conformed to the existing rules, and that radiation levels were lower than that from a microwave oven, a neon light, and radio and television transmitters.

The court agreed with Lesnikov, and ordered MTS to dismantle the tower within four months.

Russian standards regarding radiofrequency radiation and electromagnetic fields already stipulated that exposure to humans should not exceed 10 microwatts per square centimetre. Professor Oleg Grigoriev believed that in cities in particular this level should be reduced to between two and three microwatts per square centimetre.

Meanwhile, Roskomnadzor, the federal supervisor of communications and information technologies, revealed it had exposed over 1,500 cases where mobile phone operators had violated these standards.

'Such complex signals as 4G may prove far more hazardous than the ones that have existed so far,' Oleg Grigoriev was quoted in the daily *Novyie Izvestia*, 'No practical research has been conducted yet. Their safety is anyone's guess. However, the current state of affairs as it is, an overwhelming majority of people just do not care.'

Grigoriev believed that mobile phone base stations over the past two years had fundamentally changed the electromagnetic situation in cities: 'Whereas 20 years ago a tiny one percent of the urban population existed in a changed electromagnetic environment, now we can say the same about 90%. The level of electromagnetic radiation has been up with the growing number of base stations.'

Russian researchers noted that the electromagnetic radiation of all the instruments that humans had created around the globe, exceeded the Earth's own geomagnetic field many millions of times. While Russian doctors acknowledged that the effects of high frequency radiation on the human body were still poorly studied, sales were booming of bracelets and stickers said to 'ward off' harmful electromagnetic radiation.

As for Russian scientists, their recommendations to the public were simple: stay at least one and a half metres away from a working TV set or a microwave, and an arm's length away from the PC monitor. Wi-Fi transmitters should be turned off at least overnight, and mobile phones used as seldom as possible.

In Britain, meanwhile, Chief Medical Officer Professor Dame Sally Davies had taken delivery of the Russian findings. Would she heed Professor Grigoriev's call?

8 Follow the Money

The Franchisee's Tale

Driving up and down the motorways of England's green and pleasant land – whether or not you are using wireless satnav - looking out of the train, the bus, you begin to notice what you suspect you are not meant to notice.

There are the microwave masts tucked away in copses, on farmland; the masts mounted on civil institutions; on schools, hospitals, churches and police stations. The O2 Airwave Tetra mast on that barn; the Vodafone GSM combined with UMTS mast above that street; the T-Mobile combined with UMTS mast above the park; the O2 GSM and T-Mobile GSM mast above that youth centre.

You begin to wonder why you are not consulted about the government's wholesale auctioning off of bandwidth and the colonisation of public spaces, and why masts are placed where they are. You begin to wonder why these masts are placed near footpaths, on common land or in full view on public rights of way. Celebrate the liberating technology! And you begin to wonder, like Dr Diana Samways, why the newer, smaller Wi-Max masts are camouflaged: as trees, lamp posts and street signs.

You begin to wonder about the microwave crossfire you live in twenty-four hours a day and the microwave radiation pulsing in your pocket, next to your heart, your kidneys, your groin.

You begin to wonder about your children. And their children. And their children's children.

'I'd made a bit of money out of the pub and a mobile phone franchise seemed like a good proposition.'

Owen (not his real name) and his family had worked hard all their lives, most recently turning around the local pub from the one with the sticky carpet and coterie of unsmiling locals everyone avoided, to the go-to hostelry in the small market town in the Welsh borders. With the right staff in place, he and his wife could have taken it easy, retired even; but work was in the blood.

One of his children told him about becoming a mobile phone franchisee: 'My first thought was, if it's so easy, why don't *you* do it?'

The answer lay in the fact that you needed £25-50,000 to get started. Armed with the cash from the pub, Owen filled in the forms online – 'I couldn't believe how easy it was' – got a positive response to his choice of territory, and set about finding premises. Within three months he'd taken out a lease on a distressed family butcher's shop and was open for business: 'It was a bonanza. This is a rural area, and kids live quite far apart. The mobile phone retailer supplied all the marketing materials and helped with publicity. We had over a hundred people here on opening day, including the mayor and the local paper.'

How difficult was it to pass due diligence?

'It wasn't difficult at all. In fact the local estate agent told me that he'd always thought the easiest thing in the world was to become an estate agent – there were no exams, no qualifications – now he reckons he should have done what I did!'

'Anyway, he bought a phone contract off me, so that's okay.'

Did Owen have any reservations?

'Only that we're waiting for the 4G mast. That will make improve the reception. But there's some opposition, like.'

Oh, really?

'People want the phones, but they don't want the mast next to them.'

Why's that?

'Cancer… but nothing's been shown.'

Was it not strange that in this world of health and safety often taken to absurd degrees, there were no legible warnings given with mobile phones, or in mobile phone shops, or during the sales process, about the consequences of pulsing microwaves into your brain?

'Well, that's up to the customer isn't it?'

'I've got a farmer friend over the border who signed up for a mast to be put up in his field: 'Best investment I ever made,' he says, 'I'm never selling that field, no way!'

*

Far from the borders of England and Wales, students in Hong Kong had forced the removal of masts from their accommodation buildings and in India the State of Rajasthan and the City of Mumbai had passed laws prohibiting the installation of microwave masts on the roofs of hospitals and schools and in playgrounds because they were 'hazardous to life'.

In India, the Kolkata cluster of widespread physiological dysfunction identified by scientists from the Netaji Subhas Chandra Bose Cancer Research Institute (NSCRI) had occurred in spite of the fact that local radiofrequency radiations levels were already lower than the safety threshold deemed safe by ICNIRP and still adhered to in many countries around the world, including Britain. How could this be?

The answer, according to Professor Sudarshan Neogi, who co-authored a pilot study on mobile phone radiation, lay in the fact that even the revised standard of 0.92 Watt per square metre at 1,800 Mhz and 0.47 Watt per square metre at 900 MHz, was only valid assuming a maximum of one hour's exposure per day. This rendered the revised standard meaningless for people living in close proximity to masts 24 hours a day:

'So, health hazards are a possibility. But our hands are tied till we can prove that the standard is indeed faulty.'

In Britain, back in 2003, with the mobile phone industry in its infancy, there were relatively few microwave masts around the country and to all intents and purposes no available epidemiological studies to suggest links between microwave radiation and physiological harm. By 2008, there were 35,000 masts and still few such studies. By 2017, there were nearly 40,000 masts across Britain. In the same year, it was estimated a further 400,00 masts would be required to bring 5G wireless internet to rural areas of Britain. It was also estimated that, because of the growing tree line, the masts would need to be as high as 80 feet.

Or, as Brian Stein observed, 'presumably trees that were capable of growing to 80 feet would have to be chopped down.'

Over the same period, in Britain the scientific silence had intensified. Dr Gerard Hyland of the Department of Physics at the University of Warwick, who had published his findings regarding the biological effects of mobile phone masts on children, trees, plants and animals in the *Lancet* and reported his findings to the Science and Technology Committee at the House of Commons in Westminster and the European Parliament, had taken early retirement from Warwick University allegedly after 'high level' pressures were brought against his work on the biological effects of electromagnetic fields.

Dr Hyland took up a post as theoretical physicist at the International Institute of Biophysics in Neuss, Germany: 'The guidelines [based on heating effects] protect us against something that isn't a problem,' he said, arguing that, as well as heat, mobile phone and mast microwaves emitted a kind of pulsing white noise that interfered with the human body in the same way that phones interfered with aeroplane or hospital equipment. 'The alive human body is an electromagnetic instrument, not just a bag of chemicals,' he added.

Dr Hyland also predicted that base station radiation could affect humans even at very low intensities. He continued to maintain that the safety thresholds regarding masts in Britain were 'wholly inadequate' and that Government and the mobile phone industry enjoyed an unhealthy relationship at the expense of the public. As he put it: 'We are the experiment.'

The proliferation of masts in Britain had continued unchecked with conspicuously few exceptions. Eileen O'Connor and her breast cancer cluster had prevailed against T-Mobile in Wishaw in 2005; in the same year, Orange had been seen off by the mothers of Goffs Oak J.M.I and Nursery School. The Undercover Epidemiologist and colleague continued their covert work and to send their findings 'up the line'.

The Government's Site Finder Mobile Phone Base Station database, set up by Ofcom for the benefit of the public after the Stewart Report in 2000, was by its own admission out of date, because the mobile phone operators who voluntarily supplied the information as to where masts were situated, had ceased to do so, in some cases as early as 2005. In response, the pressure group Mast Sanity monitored the locations of masts and exposed the frequent lack of consultation and in many cases lack of planning permission.

In Britain, it seemed, this was still an industry more powerful than the regulators and the science whose findings it lagged behind.

But in Britain there was one industry more powerful.

The Insurance Underwriter

'Yes, there is one industry more powerful than the mobile phone industry – insurance.'

'S-J' was a senior underwriter in the London Insurance Market, based at Lloyd's, a world leader in specialist risk insurance and reinsurance. Lloyd's underwrites many kinds of risk for the dominant industries on earth – IT, defence, aviation, shipping, energy, manufacturing – industries without which the free movement of goods and services cannot take place, and we would not be able to live in our world as we do.

Recently, 'S-J''s underwriting agency had been reviewing liability cover indemnifying mobile phone operators against health damage claims by customers: 'We have bright young emerging risk researchers, and they are not only turning up some worrying things in scientific and actuarial terms, they are actually changing their personal habits.'

Where early examples of litigation such as the Reynard and Debra Wright cases in America had proved inconclusive, the Marcolini judgement in Italy, the MacDonald judgement in Australia and the settlement by Partner in Israel were tipping points. In common with other underwriting agencies, 'S-J' had concluded that the reinsurance of mobile operators was a bad business risk.

'We see this as a potential long-tail scenario,' she said, referring to the phenomenon whereby the volume of claims was such that insolvency threatened, as had happened with asbestosis in America with catastrophic results for Lloyd's in the 1980s.

Why not just put up reinsurance rates?

'We don't feel there is sufficient evidence that the mobile phone industry is willing or able to adjust existing radiation safety levels,' she said, and cited the work of Professor Lennart Hardell.

The warnings buried in the small print in mobile phone manufacturers' instructions had been drafted by lawyers concerned to protect the operators against class actions. Was this why Vodafone had dumped its holding in Verizon?

'I couldn't comment on that,' she conceded however that, as usual, British and mainland European reinsurers looked to America's lead.

'Do you use a mobile?'

'Yes, as little as possible.'

'Next to your head?'

'God, no!'

Lloyd's of London (2010): *"The danger with EMF is that, like asbestos, the exposure insurers face is underestimated and could grow exponentially and be with us for many years."* Lloyd's syndicates refuse to cover claims linked with RF radiation.

'S-J', it seemed, was very much in the business of being forewarned. In the spring of 2014, it was revealed that the reinsurance giant Swiss Re had warned of large losses from the 'unforeseen consequences' of electromagnetic frequencies. Swiss Re was a Fortune 500 company and the news that it was forecasting a raft of claims and significant liability losses sent tremors through the insurance industry.

*

In its SONAR Emerging Risks report, which covered risks that could 'impact the insurance industry in the future', the Emerging Risks team at Swiss Re categorised the impact of health claims related to electromagnetic fields (EMFs) as 'high'. Again, it acknowledged recent reports of courts ruling in favour of claimants who had experienced health damage from mobile 'phones, and also stated that anxiety over risks related to EMFs was 'on the rise'.

The document stated that whilst the majority of the topics covered in its pages were of 'medium impact', health issues associated with EMFs sat in the highest impact category. Other topics discussed include the dangers of cyber attacks, power blackouts, workplace safety and Big Data – all of which it stated were exacerbated by so-called 'smart' metering programmes.

Swiss Re defined Emerging Risks as 'newly developing or changing risks that are difficult to quantify and could have a major impact on society and insurance industry'. By placing EMFs in the 'High' potential impact-zone, it was suggesting that there may be potentially 'high financial, reputational and/or regulatory impacts or significant stakeholder concern' in the next 10 years or more.

The Swiss Re report highlighted how 'Big Utilities' and 'Big Telecom' were combined in a joint venture to convince the world that low-level chronic microwave radiation exposure was safe – even when thousands of independent peer-reviewed studies said it was not.

'If a direct link between EMF to differ and human health problems were established,' the report went on, *'it would open doors for new claims and could ultimately lead to large losses under product liability covers. Liability rates would likewise rise.'*

Swiss Re (2013): "*Over the last decade, the spread of wireless devices has accelerated enormously. ... This development has increased exposure ... If a direct link [to health effects] ... were established, it would open doors for new claims and could ultimately lead to large losses ...*"

Bermuda Re, in its casualty catastrophe modelling, likewise cited cell phones as a potential cause of *'the next asbestos'*.

The Austrian insurance company AUVA commissioned experts to assess biological effects of mobile phone radiation. Non-thermal effects were observed: "*... the demonstrated effects, should not even have occurred, according to the strictly thermal interaction mechanism that would have been covered by current exposure guidelines*".

One by one, the most powerful industries on earth were beginning to have second thoughts when it came to the joint-venture between 'Big Utilities' and 'Big Telecom.'

*

In the United States, Elizabeth Barris was a film maker whose electrosensitivity she believed had been triggered by mobile phone use, forcing her to move house repeatedly and at one point sleep every night for seven months in her car. She was part of a citizen's group which had lobbied Washington for better protective measures for cell phones, after which Motorola (who had produced the first commercial cell phone) had started printing warnings for children to keep phones away from their lower abdomens (i.e their reproductive organs) and pregnant women to keep away from their abdomens (i.e unborn fetuses).

Ms Barris and others had published a paper for the lay person on the science behind the non-thermal effects of radio frequency radiation, which had helped initiate a legislative bill to bring warnings about the health risks to the wider public: the bill had been approved in four states. She was also suing utilities giants Pacific Gas & Electric, and Edison, and had won three out of three hearings so far.

In Britain, public bodies charged with a duty of care, as ever, lagged behind.

'Letter of Notice Served on Mr Richard Adams'

'European Economic and Social Committee (EESC) Member'

'Foreign and Commonwealth Office of UK Government'

'18th February, 2015'

'Letter of Notice holding EESC member Richard Adams personally accountable for betraying public trust by ignoring evidence on the hazards of RF/EMF.'

'The Radiation Research Trust is calling for Mr Adams's appointment or re-appointment as a member of the European Economic and Social Committee (EESC) to be terminated due to his serious breach of duty and faith as a member of the EESC.'

'The Radiation Research Trust also calls for the annulment of the EESC counter-opinion and for the original opinion to be reconsidered.'

'This letter of notice is issued by the UK Radiation Research Trust in support of millions of people estimated to be between 22,000,000 and 37,000,000 throughout Europe who are currently suffering with electromagnetic hypersensitivity due to exposure to the proliferation of mobile phones, DECT cordless phones, cordless baby monitors, phone masts, Wi-Fi, smart meters and the smart grid.'

'Mr Adams instigated the counter-opinion at the EESC TEN session on electrosensitivity on 21st January, 2015 and failed to disclose his conflicts of interests which is a breach of good conduct.'

'This letter will be held on record for future reference to enable members of the public to demonstrate that information, research and reports on EMF health effects, along with details highlighting the conflicts of interests for some members from the Scientific Committee on Emerging and Newly Identified Health Risks (SCENIHR) were presented to Mr Adams before the vote for the counter-opinion on electrosensitivity EESC/TEN on 21st January, 2015.'

'We therefore wish to inform Mr Adams that we are now from today, 18th February, 2015 putting him on notice to hold him responsible for that vote's outcome. Henceforth, we will deem that Mr Adams is aware of the effects this technology is having on members of the population due to the information that we and others provided him with before the vote and future actions will have to be judged in the light of that knowledge.'

'Mr Adams was challenged over serious conflicts of interest during the EESC Plenary Session due to his (undisclosed) stakeholder position with RWE AG, one of Europe's five leading electricity and gas companies. He is also a trustee for the Charity Sustainability First (a fact that was also undisclosed at that time). Both enterprises have a vested interest in smart grid and smart meters that rely on wireless radiofrequency technology.'

'The UK Radiation Research Trust, doctors, scientists and NGOs throughout Europe expressed concerns directly to Mr Adams before that vote over the detrimental impacts wireless technology is having on millions of people who are currently suffering with electrosensitivity throughout Europe, causing damage to health and the rights to work and live in society.'

'Many people living with EHS are denied their basic human rights leading to social exclusion and disruption and destruction to family life in many cases. The adopted counter-opinion also ignores **children's rights** as they are forced to attend schools polluted by

Wi-Fi radiation and not given adequate warnings associated with the precautionary approach for children using mobile phones or other wireless technologies, thus preventing the course of Justice.'

'Mr Adams ignored such information and refused to accept that wireless technology is in any way responsible for these risks. He was not prepared to engage in dialogue of any kind and resorted to using slanderous language with regards to the work of esteemed doctors and scientists such as Professor Lennart Hardell and the BioInitiative Working Group related to biological risk.'

*

In May, 2015, 190 scientists from thirty-nine nations submitted an appeal to the UN and World Health Organisation for stronger protective exposure guidelines regarding microwave radiation and electromagnetic fields in the face of increasing evidence of risk. The World Health Organisation had hitherto continued to ignore its own safety guidelines as set down by the International Agency for Research on Cancer, in favour of those propounded by ICNIRP. The International EMF Scientist Appeal called on the UN and WHO to limit EMF exposures and educate the public more effectively about the dangers of EMFs and microwave radiation, especially to children and pregnant women.

Brian Stein's Diary, Spring 2015

Started to experience further unusual sensations in the bowel and colon. After periods of time in high EMFs need to go to the lavatory immediately and frequently. After some reflection, thought it was time to make another appointment with the doctor and brace myself for further bewilderment by the medical profession.

Brian Stein's Diary, 13 June 2015

Professor Oleg Grigoriev visited London in June 2015. We asked if he would lecture to a small group of invited guests to hear

Russia's latest findings and thoughts. We invited Public Health England, MPs and the press. The lecture took place at Friends House in London, and can be seen on the RRT website.

The MPs who responded could not make the date. The two press who responded did not turn up on the day, and Public Health England 'could not find anyone' who could attend on that day.

Professor Grigoriev concluded in his speech that:

EMFs cause cancer.

EMFs damage the central nervous system.

EMFs cause electrical sensitivity (ES).

ES is not psychosomatic.

The effects of non-ionizing radiation are the same as ionizing radiation in slow motion.

He explained the Russian conversation with the World Health Organisation, who when he asked why they had not included the Russian research in its evaluation of the dangers of EMFs, was told this was because it was not published in English.

Professor Grigoriev offered to have the sixty most important Russian research papers translated into English for WHO.

What was their response, we asked him?

They were very cool on the idea.

It seemed that the WHO did not want any more papers that proved EMFs caused cancer given that their stance had been exactly the opposite of this.

Why? We asked. Was this because the science was not good, or because it showed EMFs cause cancer?

He diplomatically shrugged his shoulders. Perhaps the WHO should be reclassified as the Western Health Organisation, he suggested. We suggested more accurately the World Mobile Protection Organisation.

More and more research is being published in the east, particularly India and China, showing that EMFs cause cancer and many other health problems. As a result of these findings, China and India have now reduced the microwave emission levels allowed in their countries to the much lower precautionary biological levels allowed by Russia, and not the thermal recommendations treated as gospel by the USA and UK.

Half of the world's population is now protected by much higher standards than those enjoyed/ endured by the west.

Meanwhile, quietly Italy, Austria, Switzerland, Luxembourg and parts of Belgium are also now adopting the stricter biological standards. All this is hardly reported in the British media.

The media are either strictly controlled by the British authorities, or there is a self-censorship simply born out of self-interest. They have a lot to lose if microwaves and wireless technology cause cancer and dementia.

A similar response was made by a former UK government minister when we discussed what was happening with standards around the world. He didn't care what was happening in Russia, China, India or indeed Italy, France or Germany. The only country that mattered was the U.S.

When they accept it causes cancer, then it will influence the UK. Not before!

*

On 2 September, 2015, twenty independent scientific organisations complained to the European Commission about the Commission's SCENIHR (Scientific Committee on Emerging and Newly-Identified Health Risks) 2015 opinion on the health effects of electromagnetic fields, on the basis that SCENIHR's data was supplied by 'industry friendly' sources:

'The SCENIHR 2015 opinion on health effects of EMF is misleading. There is evidence that clearly establishes that there are many potential negative health effects and health hazards: brain tumours, cancer, neurodegenerative diseases, damage on fetuses and stress related diseases, as communicated to the Commission by the BioInitiative group.'

'The SCENIHR report ignores the scientific evidence of health risks from levels of exposure to electromagnetic fields that practically everybody is increasingly exposed to, including small children, in most countries in Europe today. It is a disservice to the people of Europe and an indirect threat to their health.'

'The 20 organisations call for an annulment of the misleading and biased SCENIHR 2015 report on EMFs and for a new balanced and independent assessment by scientists without ties to the industry concerned about the outcome of the opinion.'

Broke Wood, Chadlington, Oxfordshire, 11 June 2015

No-one knows what Jenny Fry had in her mind that day she went down to the woods, but the 15 year-old had already left letters for her parents at their home in Chadlington saying she couldn't cope with her allergies from Wi-Fi any more. In the two and a half years since the symptoms started, the headaches, the tiredness and the bladder problems had got worse and worse whenever she went near a wireless router.

Her parents, Charles and Debra, were sympathetic and removed wireless routers from the family home. But the Wi-Fi at Chipping Norton School, where Jenny was a student, remained on.

Jenny was a diligent student, according to her mother, but the symptoms she was suffering meant she started absenting herself from classes so that she could work further away from the school's Wi-Fi.

The school's response had been to put her in detention in a room with Wi-Fi. Her mother had already had a heated exchange with teachers, and taken information about EHS into school to show the headmaster, Simon Duffy. Mr Duffy's response was that there was just as much information to show that Wi-Fi was safe.

Jenny Fry was found some time later hanging from a tree. One of the last things she did was text a friend on her mobile phone - the very technology that had made her life unbearable.

Brian Stein's Diary, 4 September 2015

Appointment with doctor. Simply explained my frequent visits to the lavatory and he suggested a blood test to check my PSA level. Blood test revealed slightly raised PSA level. Doctor suggested further PSA test in a month's time.

Brian Stein's Diary, 22 October 2015

Another blood test. PSA level slightly raised again.

Brian Stein's Diary, 20 November 2015

Doctor considered monitoring PSA level. Did not think it was an issue – only slightly raised – but continues to monitor.

Brian Stein's Diary, 28 November 2015

Small bleed when peeing after a period in a Wi-Fi environment.

Brian Stein's Diary, 30 November 2015

'Phone appointment with Doctor. Mentioned slight blood show two days before. He suggests some tests.

Brian Stein's Diary, 9 December 2015

Queen's Hospital. Camera into bowel. Enlarged prostate but nothing to worry about. Bowel clear.

Brian Stein's Diary, 16 December 2015

Queen's Hospital. Ultrasound. All appears to be okay.

Brian Stein's Diary, 21 December 2015

Prostate biopsy.

Brian Stein's Diary, 31 December 2015

Results of biopsy. Prostate cancer. Grade 7, so action required.

Brian Stein's Diary, 7 January 2016

Queen's Hospital. MRI Scan.

Brian Stein's Diary, 19 January 2016

Results of scan. Cancer not spread beyond prostate. Removal of prostate very difficult because of the size of the prostate and growing into the bladder. Hospital cannot provide a Wi-Fi-free environment for recovery. Radiotherapy recommended. How will this affect an ES person?

Brian Stein's Diary, 29 January 2016

More severe bleeding after spending long period in Wi-Fi environment. Continued to bleed for a few days.

Brian Stein's Diary, 19 February 2016

Started hormone treatment with a view to shrinking the prostate and starting radiotherapy in the summer. Oh joy!

No follow-up by researchers after being exposed in their tests! Have those claiming to be ES been damaged, or have a higher incidence of cancer?

Brian Stein's Diary, 7 October 2016

Visited Rosmani – House of Prayer, to organise ES-UK conference. Looked great on the website. No Wi-Fi as a principle. In the countryside. Ideal. Found a wireless mast on the next door school grounds only a few hundred yards away.

Brian Stein's Diary, 13 October 2016

Attended conference at the Royal Society in London on the 'Bradford Hill' precautionary principle. Met up with Lennart Hardell, who is very concerned at how the authorities are ignoring the research.

The NTP (National Toxicology Program) presented, but on the chemical research approach, they were not involved with the microwave research. We asked them about timescales for the publication of NTP report findings. Their comment was 'it was way above their pay grade. It was now with the politicians.' Worrying.

*

Charles and Debra Fry, the parents of Jenny Fry, had attended the inquest into the suicide of their daughter, which they believed her school could have prevented. Headmaster Simon Duffy disagreed: 'Just like many other public spaces, Chipping Norton School does have Wi-Fi installed to enable us to operate effectively,' he told the inquest. 'The governors are content that the installed equipment complies with the relevant regulations and will ensure this continues to be the case.'

Coroner Darren Salter's verdict did not include factors relating to EHS on the grounds that no medical notes existed to prove that Jenny had suffered from the condition. Jenny's parents were not content to leave things there. They made contact with ES-UK's Dr. Erica Mallery-Blythe. They successfully lobbied for fifteen minutes with the Prime Minister, a resident of Chipping Campden, and

Dr. Mallery-Blythe accompanied Debra Fry on the occasion. They raised a petition calling for greater awareness of EHS and the removal of wireless technologies from nurseries and schools. As Debra Fry put it: 'I am on the warpath to protect our children and get justice for Jenny.'

*

In April, 2016, the Israeli TV documentary 'How We Are Killing Ourselves – Wireless Radiation' concentrated on ES and Wi-Fi in schools and had the highest ratings of the day. The programme suggested that as many as 800,000 in Israel – 10% of the population - suffered from varying levels of ES and described the situation as 'an epidemic'. Participants included Dafna Tachover, a leading campaigner to raise awareness of the physiological effects of Wi-Fi, and two Israeli government 'experts' who admitted that, contrary to what they had recently testified to Israel's Supreme Court, the current industry thermal safety standards were 'irrelevant'.

Shortly after the programme was broadcast, the Mayor of Haifa, Israel's third largest city, Yona Yahav, ordered all Wi-Fi to be removed from schools and replaced with hard-wired internet: 'When there is a doubt, when it comes to our children, there is no doubt,' he declared. Other cities in Israel were expected to follow suit.

*

In May, 2016, *Microwave News* in New York City announced that the shortly-to-be-released US National Toxicology Program two-year study on the health effects of non-thermal wireless radiation confirmed the presence of brain and heart tumours in rats exposed to levels of radiation even lower than that those currently declared safe by cell phone operators: the animal exposure levels in the study being comparable to those of heavy cell phone users.

The report concluded that cell phone radiation presented a carcinogenic threat to humans. The NTP was poised to make a public announcement to this effect and discussions were already under way among federal agencies as to how best to inform the public of the dangers.

'Given the widespread global usage of mobile communications among users of all ages, even a very small increase in the incidence of disease resulting from exposure to radio frequency radiation could have broad implications for public health,' NTP researchers stated in a report issued alongside the study.

The news of the NTP findings was greeted as 'a paradigm shift' and 'good science' by Dr Otis Brawley, chef medical officer of the American Cancer Society. Retired NTP researcher Ron Melnick had worked on the study. He told the *Wall Street Journal*: 'Where people were saying there's no risk, I think this ends that kind of statement.'

David Carpinter, Director of the School of Public Health at State University, New York in Albany, said the study 'won't end the debate, but I can't imagine anything more credible than an NTP report.'

Professor Dariusz Leszczynski in Finland agreed: 'The National Toxicology Program's study should have been done a long time ago,' he said, 'before cell phones were commercially introduced on the market. This is a typical toxicology study aimed at determining the safety of a radiation-emitting gadget.'

*

Dr Sarah Starkey was an independent neuroscientist and environmental health researcher in London. Starkey had read and analysed the 2012 'findings' of the Advisory Group on Non-Ionising Radiation (AGNIR), which was the official source of advice on radio frequency electromagnetic fields to Public Health England. In the opinion of Starkey and many others, it was imperative in the interests of good science and the public health that such reports were independent of wireless industry influence.

Yet, her analysis showed that, at the time of the report's writing, the chairman of AGNIR was also chair of the ICNIRP standing committee on epidemiology, and that as of 2016 six members of AGNIR and three members of Public Health England or its parent the Department of Health, were or had been part of ICNIRP. This was a misleading report which to the expert eye revealed a conflict of interests, was conspicuous by its omissions, and the conclusions of which did not reflect the full body of scientific evidence.

As Dr Starkey put it: *'How can AGNIR report that the scientific literature contains evidence of harmful effects under the current guidelines when several of them are responsible for those guidelines?'* **(see link to Starkey analysis in Appendix 6)**

*

In June, 2017, Brian Stein was invited to speak at the Glastonbury Science Symposium, part of the world-famous music festival of the same name. Out of 175,000 attendees, he was probably the only person wearing a tie.

Brian Stein's Diary, 29 June 2017

Glastonbury Science Symposium. Friendly audience, many ES. Very few if any needed converting. The presentation can be viewed on You Tube. Google 'Glastonbury Science Symposium Brian Stein'. Enjoy!

Brian Stein's Diary, 29 January 2018

The National Toxicology Program announces the overdue study will be published in February 2018 and peer-reviewed at the end of March 2018.

Brian Stein's Diary, 4 February 2018

The doubt has started.

Some scientists are saying the National Toxicology Program shows a link between cell phones and cancer. Other 'experts' are saying it doesn't. Here we go again.

Jeff Shurer, Director of the US Food & Drug Administration says 'these findings should not be extrapolated to humans. The findings are mostly equivocal or ambiguous.'

The spin has started.

I wonder what would have been said if he had said the same thing about the tobacco experiments on rats and mice not being relevant for humans, or indeed the drug industry ignoring their results on animals because they should not be extrapolated to humans!

The Food & Drug Administration funds the ultimate research to find the truth. When it finds the truth, it backtracks.

Obviously not the results they wanted or expected.

As more independent studies continued to emerge showing the toxic effects of wireless technology and mobile phone radiation levels on rats and mice, the doubt and spin were deployed incrementally. *The Times* headline of 5 February, 2018 with regard to the National Toxicology Program, read: '*Mobile phones 'do not cause cancer'*.

As Brian Stein, in common with many others, observed: *However in the report it says they did find tumours!*

Brian Stein's Diary, 25 February 2018

Following the NTP study, the Ramazzini Institute in Bologna, Italy, releases major new animal study linking radio frequency radiation to cancer. It is the largest ever animal study on low-level radiation from mobile phone masts and confirms the NTP study that both low-level (masts and Wi-Fi) and high-level microwave emissions (phone to head) cause cancerous tumours in rats exposed to environmental levels of radio frequency radiation...

These findings will cause alarm with the authorities so one can expect serious doubts to be raised by ICNIRP, Public Health England and the authorities empowered supposedly to protect our health. What these studies show that will be most alarming is that, like passive smoking, you can get cancer from mobile phone technology even if you do not use it.

Brian Stein's Diary, 2 April 2018

Expert panel following the National Toxicology Program peer review says 'clear evidence of cancer.' They voted to strengthen the conclusions that cell phone radiation causes health effects: 'Clear evidence of carcinogenity of the heart. Some evidence of carcinogenity of the brain. In addition, 'statistically significant' increased numbers of tumours in prostate, pituitary and adrenal glands, the pancreas and liver.'

The UK Radiation Research Trust complained to IPSO (the Independent Press Standards Organisation) about the accuracy of the *Times* headline of 5 February. The complaint was rejected. When the RRT appealed against the logic of the rejection, the appeal was rejected.

As Brian Stein wrote in his diary: *Therefore IPSO ruled that these comments validated the Times headline rather than the (NTP) study and the peer review that concluded 'clear evidence of cancer'.*

We live in a world of authorised 'fake news'.

Cancer Research UK, a long-time denier of links between wireless radiation, mobile phones and cancer, commented on the NTP findings that it was *'unlikely that phones could increase the risk of brain tumours or any cancer, but it cannot be ruled out.'*

There were places that spin could not reach. On 21 June, 2018, the UK science journalist Geoffrey Lean in the mass circulation

Daily Mail newspaper cited the statement by Professor Anthony Miller of Toronto University and a former Director of Canada's National Cancer Institute's Epidemiology Unit, that W-Fi *'should not be allowed in schools.'*

Lean also cited examples of the precautionary principle being introduced in kindergartens and schools in Israel, Germany, Spain, Belgium, France, Cyprus and Polynesia – adding: *'Here in Britain, by contrast, there is only complacency and inaction – despite authoritative early warnings of trouble ahead'* (a reference to Sir William Stewart's report of nearly two decades earlier.

Brian Stein's Diary, June 2018

Russia has produced many papers on the dangers of microwaves, concluding that Western standards do not meet basic hygiene requirements.

Most of these papers have been ignored in the West as they are written in Russian. Now that they are being translated, they are being rubbished as 'fake news' as the West rolls out 5G.

Even the evidence from western countries is ignored as the science of mobile communications is controlled by the industry... and not by any consideration of the science showing harmful effects, particularly to vulnerable groups, i.e children.

'Mobile Communications and Public Health' edited by Marko Markov and published by CRC Press, Taylor and Francis Group, outlines much of the Russian research and why there should be a moratorium on 5G.

*

In November, 2018, *The Times* of London reported that Gary Taylor, the proprietor of Babeek, a luxury *'organic'* nursery furniture business in Birmingham - *'All our furniture is designed to be safe as well as beautiful'* – intended to produce a £1,500 'Intelligent Cot' with a built-in iPad.

Mr Taylor was reported as stating he created the cot after having trouble getting his daughter Graysie to sleep – his solution being to use the iPad to play white noise to her: 'I know people put their kids in front of the TV in the morning,' Mr Taylor was quoted as saying, 'is that safe? I was thinking that if they could put it in the cot it could be a lot safer.'

'Kids are stuck on their computers. That's the way the generation is going. I'm giving people what they want.'

At the time of writing, Babeek had not replied to an enquiry from these authors and the proposed product was not offered on the company's website.

Brian Stein's Diary, 8 March 2019

Lloyd's insurers are refusing to cover 5G Wi-Fi illness. Ask yourself why, if it is impossible to be damaged by non-ionising radiation, insurers would pass up the billions of pounds available to insure against something that ICNIRP, Public Health England and the industry say is impossible?

Brian Stein's Diary, March 2019

Since the fall out from the National Toxicology Program and Ramazzini studies showing EMFs causing cancer in rats and mice, the authorities have taken an unusual, but effective step: announcing that rats and mice are not human, so of no relevance.

Then why did the Food & Drug Administration in the US give US $25 million to carry out these studies if they were not relevant? Why is ICNIRP trying to repeat them with rats and mice in Japan?

I worked all my life in the food industry. Before I retired the industry had the largest product recall in its history. Food – pies and ready meals – were found accidentally to contain 'Sudan 1', an ingredient that had been added to Worcester Sauce and supplied throughout the industry.

Sudan 1 had been found in a study to be carcinogenic to rats and mice at thousands of times higher than the dose in the food chain, but after constant newspaper comment about how disgraceful this was, the Food Standards Agency recalled all food containing the ingredient.

Similarly, my wife is a research scientist in the drugs industry, researching a cure for asthma sufferers.

Any drug found to be carcinogenic to rats and mice in trials is immediately stopped and research ended.

If a foodstuff, or a drug, had failed toxicity testing with rats and mice, the authorities, the press, the politicians, the public would not allow it to be used on the public.

When the same is true of mobile phones and Wi-Fi, all of a sudden research using rats and mice is not relevant. Someone should be before the courts for this double standard.

Now, 5G will be a massive new trial, on humans, and we already know it increases the incidence of cancer in rats and mice.

No wonder Lloyd's of London will not insure against damage from microwave radiation.

We are taking advice from a small, self-appointed circle of insiders who reject all research showing harm, and who set safety limits.

Should we now ignore cancer in rats and mice for research into foodstuffs and new drugs because they are not human experiments? Why is the press not investigating this double standard, instead of simply accepting this new paradigm as fact?

Brian Stein's Diary, 3 June 2019

Microwave News reports colorectal cancer is soaring among young adults. Epidemiologist De-Kun Li suggests with young people carrying smartphones in trousers, the phone is closest to the rectum and the distal colon, the sites of the largest increases in cancer.

Brian Stein's Diary, 20 July 2019

'Birth of Smart Nappy'. Pampers launch in the US that transmits to an app when the baby is wet. 'The days of smelling your tot's butt are gone,' says Dr Ali Khan, a public health expert at University of Nebraska. (Not sure how it transmits, but next to new-born baby's private parts).

Brian Stein's Diary, 22 July 2019

Steep rise in young people suffering from bowel cancer. A study in the US has found the rate among people under 50 has risen from one in ten to more than one in eight in just eleven years.

The same trend has been identified in the UK. Younger adults are being diagnosed with more aggressive growths.

A study of 20 European countries, including the UK, has found that the number of 20 to 39-year-olds who have been diagnosed with bowel cancer increased by 6% every year between 2008 and 2016. Asha Kaur, head of policy at Bowel Cancer UK, said every year more than 2,500 people under 50 are diagnosed with bowel cancer, a 48% increase in the number of cases since 2004.

(With mobile phones kept in pockets, the bowel is particularly sensitive to EMFs, and research shows that phones kept in pockets with metal (coins or keys) results in emission levels above the guidelines).

*

In July, 2019, two states in North America, New Hampshire and Oregon, commissioned major studies into the public health effects of wireless radiation from 5G technology.

In New Hampshire, House Bill 522 signed by Governor Sununu included the following statement:

'Fifth generation, or 5G, wireless technology is intended to greatly increase device capability and connectivity but also may pose *significant risk to humans, animals and the environment due to increased radiofrequency radiation exposure. The purpose of the study is to examine the advantages and risks associated with 5G technology, with a focus on its environmental impact and potential health effects, particularly on children, foetuses, the elderly, and those with existing health compromises.'*

Membership of the commission would be a cross-section of the public and private sectors of the community. The New Hampshire bill cut to the chase with the following questions among others:

'Why the insurance industry recognises wireless radiation as a leading risk and has placed exclusions in their policies not covering damages caused by the pathological effects of electromagnetic radiation?'

'Why do cell phone manufacturers have in the legal section within the device saying keep the phone at least 5mm from the body?'

'Why have 1,000s of peer-reviewed studies, including the recently published U.S Toxicology Program 16-year $25 million study, that are showing a wide range of statistically significant DNA damage, brain and heart tumours, infertility and so many other ailments, been ignored by the Federal Communication Commission (FCC)?'

'Why are the FCC-sanctioned guidelines for public exposure to wireless radiation based only on the thermal effect on the temperature of the skin and do not account for the non-thermal, non-ionizing, biological effects of wireless radiation?'

'Why have more than 220 of the world's leading scientists signed an appeal to the WHO and the United Nations to protect public health from wireless radiation and nothing has been done?'

'Why have the cumulative biological damaging effects of ever-growing numbers of pulse signals riding on the back of electromagnetic sine waves not been explored, especially as the world embraces the Internet of Things, meaning all devices being connected by electromagnetic waves, and the exploration of the number of such pulse signals that will be created by the implementation of 5G technology?'

The commission expected to present its final report on or before 1 November 2020.

In Oregon, Senate Bill 283 proposed:

'An act relating to exposure to radiation in schools in this state; and declaring an emergency.'

'The Oregon Health Authority shall:'

'Review peer-reviewed, independently funded scientific studies of the health effects of exposure to microwave radiation, particularly exposure that results from the use of wireless network technologies in schools or similar environments.'

'The Department of Education shall develop recommendations to schools in this state for practices and alternative technologies that would reduce students' exposure to microwave radiation that the review described in subsection (1) of this section identifies as harmful.'

'This 2019 Act being necessary for the immediate preservation of the public peace, health and safety, an emergency is declared to exist, and this 2019 Act takes effect on its passage.'

Brian Stein's Diary, July, August, September 2019

Planning for the Radiation Research Trust conference in London in September. The major independent scientists from around the world are presenting the findings of the National Toxicology Program in the US (the first time in the UK) and the Ramazzini Institute study in Italy (so far unreported in the UK) and the implications they have for the roll-out of 5G.

Central London, 28 September 2019

The Radiation Research Trust 'Radiation Health 2019: Get the Facts' International Conference, chaired by Brian Stein with the assistance of Dr Erica Mallery-Blythe, was the first on this scale in the UK and unprecedented in the range and depth of its speakers.

The Hallam Conference Centre – formerly the offices of the General Medical Council – saw the coming together of leading independent scientists and researchers from around the world.

Dr Dimitris Papadopoulos from the University of Athens, Greece showed why his theory on the mechanism of the actions of EMFs (Electromagnetic Fields) on cells was considered the most valid. His experiments were among the first to show the damaging effects of microwaves and other man-made EMFs on DNA and reproduction.

Dr Papadopoulos reminded the conference that 'All living organisms have an EM (Electromagnetic) nature and have since the beginning of evolution lived in an EM environment.' He illustrated the fragmentation of DNA in the ovarian cells of insects from exposure to man-made mobile telephony fields, even for only six minutes a day, and rubbished ICNIRP's ignoring of the non-thermal and non-ionising effects and their attitude that 'If we can't measure it, it doesn't exist.'

He pointed out that independent peer-reviewed studies into these effects recorded measurable results in between 60% to 98% of cases.

Dr Papadopoulos concluded with a series of suggestions echoing Sir William Stewart's precautionary principle and the National Toxicology Program and Ramazzini Institute findings, and called for an urgent reconsideration of current safety standards.

Professor Martin Pall, Professor Emeritus of Biochemistry and Basic Medical Sciences at Washington State University, USA, had received 9 international honours for research in Environmental Medicine and authored 102 professional publications.

In a demolition of the mobile industry's 'safety' guidelines, Professor Pall demonstrated in the true sense of the word exactly why the industry called him 'alarmist'. He began by describing how each of the cells in our bodies is calcium-low and surrounded by a membrane, and each membrane opens up channels. EMFs open up these channels and introduce a far greater volume of calcium ions, which, in Professor Pall's words, 'wreak havoc.'

By Professor Pall's calculations, citing Coulomb's Law, the mobile industry guidelines exposed bioactivity in humans to EMFs that were 'as much as 7.2 million times too high.' He described a recent ICNIRP paper as 'total fiction'.

Professor Pall acknowledged that therapeutic effects of EMFs were appropriate under suitable controlled medical conditions. The irony was that, if the mobile industry could not acknowledge the destructive effects on human bioactivity, they could not acknowledge the therapeutic ones.

The ICNIRP standards 'don't work and have been passively adopted around the world.'

Occupational exposure to non-thermal microwave radiation was at least five times higher than general public exposure. The fact that industry guidelines only measured heating and not non-thermal exposure was 'a huge problem'.

Professor Pall went on to describe further areas in which the safety guidelines failed:

Lower fertility.

Neurological/neuropsychiatric effects.

DNA cellular damage.

Cancers.

Cardiac effects, including sudden cardiac death – 'a major issue'.

More than 197 studies, Professor Pall pointed out, demonstrated the above and more 'and cannot be shown to be flawed.' The 'smarter' the device, the more pulses and therefore the greater danger:

'5G,' he told the conference, 'is a huge issue and is completely ignored by the industry safety guidelines, that only cite average intensity that can be ten billion times lower.' The industry physics was 'fatally flawed and inconsistent with real physics' – placing 4G and 5G antennae all over communities would be 'an extraordinarily dangerous combination.'

5G would also be 'a highly unpredictable situation.' The industry safety guidelines were 'bogus, fraudulent and totally unscientific. They don't protect us one iota.'

Professor Pall concluded his presentation with 'My worst nightmares,' adding that, in some cases, they were 'already far along.'

With regard to male fertility in particular, he cited low fertility rates in Switzerland, Finland and Denmark and predicted increased infertility in the most densely-microwaved populations, especially in Asia: 'We are taking risks,' he said, 'of the sort that no rational society on earth should take.' The effects within even two or three years would be 'absolutely stunning. 5G will push countries off a reproductive cliff.'

The neurological and neuropsychiatric effects of an insufficiently regulated 5G could in his judgement produce 'a crash in effective brain function in five to six years – utter chaos.' Increases in early onset Alzheimer's and other dementias were likely, as was an 'epidemic' in autism. The damage to our DNA and gene pool, to cardiac function, the ecology in general, could not be overestimated.

'5G,' Professor Pall stated flatly, 'is a threat equal to nuclear annihilation and must be stopped.'

Professor Lennart Hardell's research had been instrumental in the Marcolini legal judgement in Italy and the classification of non-thermal microwave radiation as a potential carcinogen, in particular the health dangers from mobile and cordless phones regarding brain tumours.

He had published more than 300 peer-reviewed papers, been awarded several scientific prizes and held positions at the Department of Oncology, Orebro University Hospital in Sweden, and the School of Public Health, University of California in Berkeley, USA.

The mobile phone operators and ICNIRP were even more afraid of Professor Hardell than they were of Professor Pall. When they attacked his research for 'lacking rigor' the independent scientific community audited his methodology and declared when it came to rigor, Hardell's was 'the gold standard'.

Professor Hardell's theme was 'What we are not told by the industry and the media.'

He showed Om P. Gandhi's slides of the human brain at 5 years, 10 years and adulthood. The progressive exposure to radiation with each evolution up to the smartphone, the antenna of which was at the base of the device, was evident on the thyroid in particular.

Professor Hardell pointed to the rise in thyroid cancers, the WHO classification of non-thermal radiation as potentially carcinogenic, the NTP and Ramazzini Institute findings and the increases in gliomas, acoustic neuromas, tinnitus and hearing difficulties.

He contrasted the rigor of these studies with papers in Australia and Sweden from ICNIRP, which he dismissed as 'lacking in verified mechanisms for radiofrequency carcinogenesis' and as such were 'Fake science... Not true... Rubbish. The opposite of the ICNIRP studies is true.'

Of the chair and vice-chair of the committee behind the ICNIRP papers, Rodney Croft and Maria Feychting, Professor Hardell said: 'This casts doubt on all literature published by these persons,' adding, 'They discredit scientific honour.'

Professor Hardell went on to describe more about how 5G would function. The signals from base stations would fly back and forth constantly, following the user. If child blocked the signal, the signal power from the base station would be increased, increasing exposure. He predicted bioactivity damage to skin, eyes, sweat glands, and general tissue.

The industry, he went on, was intensively lobbying governments over the roll out: yet 5G would be 'impossible' in some countries because of the limit to the size of emissions in exclusion zones around masts and base stations.

He cited Dr Sarah Starkey's expose of how industry-sponsored studies cross-quoted each other to present a unified version of 'findings' that was increasingly at odds with the scientific facts: 'It means the media doesn't pay enough attention to this problem.'

'We should have ethical permission,' he went on, 'for people who are going to be exposed to 5G. There should be the possibility of legal action.'

'Thirteen persons in ICNIRP,' he concluded, 'make decisions for the whole world – as opposed to 250 persons who have signed the independent scientific declaration.'

Dr. Ron Melnick was an award-winning senior toxicologist for 28 years in the US National Toxicology Program (NTP). He led the design of the NTP's Toxicology and Carcinogenesis Studies of Cell Phone Radiofrequency Radiation in Rodents. He had also served a year at the White House Office of Science and Technology Policy, on the World Health Organisation's panel which classified RFR as a possible carcinogen and was an emeritus fellow of the Collegium Ramazzini.

In the first UK presentation of the NTP findings, Dr. Melnick showed, as Brian Stein put it in his introduction, 'why ICNIRP are panicking about his research.' He described the methodology employed and the spectrum of findings relating to evidence of lesions, cancers in the heart, brain and prostate and effects on DNA, the heart muscle and fertility. He also suggested that the classification in some cases – 'Clear evidence', 'Some evidence' and 'Equivocal' had been toned down.

He suggested flaws in the 2011-13 International Agency for Research on Cancer (IARC) study compared with the NTP study and supported the findings of the Ramazzini Institute, particularly with regard to the increased evidence of heart schwanommas (tumours).

Dr. Melnick reiterated the recommendations of previous speakers when it came to what the public needed to know and was not being told. With five billion cell phones in the world, he said, the Specific Absorption Rate (SAR) in humans needed to be properly quantified in terms of risk. The precautionary principles should be promoted by the regulatory authorities: 'No technology regarding 5G,' he concluded, 'should be assumed to be safe without further testing.'

Dr. Andrea Vornoli was a researcher at the Cesare Maltoni Cancer Research Centre of the Ramazzini Institute in Bologna, Italy. His work was in the fields of Toxicology, Molecular Biology, Nutritional Biochemistry and Cancer Research. In the first major UK presentation of the Ramazzini Institute studies into long-term ELF (Extremely Low Frequency) and EMF exposure and mobile 'phone radio frequency exposure, he described the research and findings that carried his name. Funders of the rearch included Children with Cancer UK and the US Environmental Health Trust.

Dr. Vornoli introduced his presentation with the credo of the Ramazzini Institute: 'It pays far more to prevent than to treat.' He described the methodology he used that led to the first Ramazzini paper in 2016, which showed 'a significant increase in carcinomas and lymphomas' from low level radiofrequency exposure in mice and rats. A second study published in 2016 again showed significant increases: the findings of the third study would be published at the end of 2019.

Dr. Vornoli's studies had exposed mice and rats to lower doses than the NTP Program, yet still found increases in brain gliomas and heart schwanommas. Like Dr. Melnick, he called for a re-evaluation of the International Agency for Research on Cancer study and noted that the IARC would include Radiofrequency radiation in its 2020-2024 research programme.

He described as 'incredible' the increase in temporal and frontal lobe timours in humans over the last decade. 5G and The Internet of Things were 'a serious risk to human, animal and environmental health.'

'There is an urgent need to review,' he said, adding that previous early warnings from the Ramazzini Institute 'had a history of being ignored.'

Dr. Peter Ohnsorge of the European Academy for Environmental Medicine, the European Cancer and Environmental Research Institute and the Robert Koch Institute in Berlin, Brian Stein, chairman of the EM Radiation Research Trust, Dr. Devra Davis, founder and president of the Environmental Health Trust and Dr. Erica Mallery-Blythe rounded off the individual presentations. A panel discussion with all speakers took questions from the media. The combined speakers received a standing ovation.

*

The independent scientists invited to peer review the National Toxicology Program findings had concluded the study showed 'clear evidence of cancer' and voted to strengthen the conclusions of the report. Nevertheless, they had come to suspect that, like the Food & Drug Administration, the National Toxicology Program leaders were downplaying the conclusions.

Were the government-funded FDA and NTP under pressure from what, by this time, like 'big oil' and 'big tobacco', had become 'big wireless'.

The roll out of 5G required for the 'Internet of Things' revealed the industry's intention to bathe communities worldwide in microwave radiation from mobile phones, cordless phones, tablets, laptop computers, desktop computers, 'smart' meters, and base stations, on a scale as never before.

All this would be implemented with minimal or no public consultation, while maintaining that wireless radiation was safe because the wireless industry and its industry-funded 'experts' said so, with any legal caveats buried in the smallest print.

By this time, it was reported that the average user spent the equivalent of one day a week online.

Then came 'Phonegate'.

San Francisco, USA, December 2019

'FeganScott Law Firm Confirms PhoneGate: New FCC-Accredited Lab Results Show Apple and Samsung Smartphone RF Radiation Levels Exceed Federal Limit'

'Third-party test results show radiation exposure exceeds five times the federal limit'

'San Francisco – December 6, 2019 – National consumer-rights law firm FeganScott consolidated its two proposed class action suits against Apple (AAPL) and Samsung Electronics (SSNLF) after independent testing from a Federal Communications Commission-accredited laboratory confirmed that radio-frequency (RF) radiation levels from popular Apple and Samsung smartphones far exceeded federal limits when the devices are used as marketed by the manufacturers.'

'Beth Fegan, managing partner of FeganScott and the attorney representing the consolidated suit, which was filed after the firm hired the industry-recognized lab, says that smartphone manufacturers must take responsibility for misleading consumers about the levels of RF radiation emitted by their smartphones when used against or in close proximity to the user's skin.'

"Apple and Samsung smartphones have changed the way we live. Adults, teenagers and children wake up to check their email or play games and do work or school exercises on their smartphones. They carry these devices in their pockets throughout the day and literally fall asleep with them in their beds," Fegan said.

"The manufacturers told consumers this was safe, so we knew it was important to test the RF radiation exposure and see if this was true," Fegan noted. "It is not true. The independent results confirm that RF radiation levels are well over the federal exposure limit, sometimes exceeding it by 500 percent, when phones are used in the way Apple and Samsung encourage us to. Consumers deserve to know the truth."

'The FCC-accredited lab tested six different brand-new smartphone models at various distances, ranging from zero to 10 millimeters to measure the amount of RF radiation released when touching or in close proximity to the body. When tested at two millimeters, the iPhone 8 and Samsung Galaxy S8 were more than twice the federal exposure limit. At zero millimeters, the iPhone 8 was five times more than the federal exposure limit, and the Samsung Galaxy S8 was more than three times the federal exposure limit.'

'The consolidated suit filed by FeganScott includes a comprehensive list of all named plaintiffs and includes the extensive FCC-accredited lab test results from all the smartphones tested: iPhone 7+, iPhone 8, iPhone XR, Galaxy S8, Galaxy S9, and Galaxy S10.'

'The test settings reflected the smartphones' actual use conditions, rather than the conditions set by manufacturers in order to produce results that appear to be safe for consumers.'

"Smartphone owners across the country deserve to know that the RF radiation levels from smartphones when touching the skin or used close to the body may be unsafe," Fegan noted. "The emails and calls from concerned consumers have increased as more research comes to light, and it is our goal to show that Apple and Samsung were aware of the alarmingly high radiation levels when their products arrived on the market."

'According to Pew Research Center, 96 percent of Americans own a cell phone, and of those, 81 percent own a smartphone. Common Sense Media, a nonprofit organization, reports that 29 percent of American teens sleep with their phones in bed with them, which makes the radiation level findings especially alarming.'

'Filed Thursday in U.S. District Court in the Northern District of California, San Francisco Division, the lawsuit seeks to represent

Apple and Samsung smartphone owners. The suit asks the court to order the defendants to pay for medical monitoring and damages.'

'FeganScott is a nationwide class-action law firm dedicated to helping consumers. The firm's partners have successfully recovered $1 billion on behalf of consumers and victims nationwide. FeganScott is committed to pursuing successful outcomes with integrity and excellence, while holding unjust parties accountable. To learn more, visit www.feganscott.com.'

Brian Stein's Diary, 10 January 2020

Approximately fifteen years ago, mobile phone manuals started to include in the small print the fact that the phone 'should be kept 0.98 inches (25mm) from the body when transmitting… including the abdomen of pregnant women and the lower abdomen of teenagers… and reduce the amount of time spent on calls.' Also that the phone should not be worn or carried on the body.'

This warning from manufacturers was not followed up by regulatory bodies or Public Health England. I wondered at the time what they knew that they were failing to communicate to the general public.

Three years ago we found out why.

The public health issue of Phonegate has revealed that many phones are exceeding the SAR (Specific Absorption Rate) threshold set at 2w/kg. The SAR is set to protect cell phone users from overheating or thermal effects. It is well-established that thermal effects can be harmful to health.

The French National Agency for Food, Environmental and Occupational Health and Safety (ANSES) report entitled 'Exposure to Radiofrequencies and Child Health' highlights that of 95 mobile phones tested in body contact positions (normal use) 90% exceeded the regulatory threshold. These results were kept secret from consumers.

French physician Dr Mark Arazi took legal action to force ANFR (the French National Frequency Agency) which manages all radio frequencies in France to make these results public. Of 21 cell phone models, 17 have been withdrawn from the market or updated as a result of Phonegate's actions.

ANFR had given notice to companies to take action to comply with legislation and in the absence of a response from two companies they proceeded to withdraw two phones from the market. Nine cell phone models are the subject of class actions/criminal complaints in France.

The ANFR data reveals that 250 cell phone models exceed the regulatory limits and must be withdrawn. These phones continue to be sold not only in France and Europe but many other countries.

Clearly, all cell phone manufacturers must have realised their phones exceeded the regulatory limits 15 years ago, and rather than making changes to comply, simply started testing emissions for SAR compliance at a distance of 25mm from the body and put this warning in the small print, while knowing that the consumer is not aware, and indeed it is virtually impossible to use a phone while it is 25mm away from the body.

This should be a bigger scandal than the diesel emission levels, but instead of government testing and informing the public, Public Health England ignores this.

Turin, January 2020

The Court of Appeal in Turin confirmed for a second time the link between a head tumour and mobile phone use.

Switzerland, February 2020

'Switzerland halts rollout of 5G over health concerns.'

'The country's environment agency has called time on the use of all new towers.'

'Switzerland, one of the world's leaders in the rollout of 5G mobile technology, has placed an indefinite moratorium on the use of its new network because of health concerns. The move comes as countries elsewhere around Europe race to upgrade their networks to 5G standards amid a furious rearguard diplomatic campaign by the US to stop them using Chinese technology provided by Huawei. Washington says the company, which is fundamental to most European networks' upgrade plans, presents a grave security risk.'

'Switzerland is relatively advanced in Europe in adopting 5G. The wealthy alpine country has built more than 2,000 antennas to upgrade its network in the last year alone, and its telecoms providers have been promising their customers' imminent 5G coverage for most of the past year. However, a letter sent by the Swiss environment agency, Bafu, to the country's cantonal governments at the end of January, has now in effect called time on the use of all new 5G towers, officials who have seen the letter told the Financial Times.'

'The agency is responsible for providing the cantons with safety criteria against which telecoms operators' radiation emissions can be judged. Under Switzerland's highly federalised structure, telecoms infrastructure is monitored for compliance and licensed by cantonal authorities, but Bern is responsible for setting the framework. Bafu has said it cannot yet provide universal criteria without further testing of the impact of 5G radiation. The agency said it was "not aware of any standard worldwide" that could be used to benchmark recommendations. "Therefore Bafu will examine exposure through adaptive [5G] antennas in depth, if possible in real-world operational conditions. This work will take some time," it said. Without the criteria, cantons are left with little option but to license 5G infrastructure according to existing guidelines on radiation exposure, which all but preclude the use of 5G except in a tiny minority of cases.'

'Several cantons have already imposed their own voluntary moratoria because of uncertainty over health risks. Swiss law on the effects of radiation from telecoms masts is broadly in line with that of European peers, but specifies the application of more stringent precautionary measures in certain cases. New 5G communications technology means individuals are exposed to more concentrated beams of non-ionising radiation, but for shorter periods. Bafu must determine which legal standards to apply to this. Swisscom, the country's largest mobile operator, said it understood "the fears that are often expressed about new technologies". "There is no evidence that antenna radiation within the limit values adversely affects human health," the company added, pointing out that 5G is run on frequencies similar to the current 4G standard, which has been subject to "several thousand studies." The company said Switzerland's regulatory limits were "10 times stricter than those recommended by the World Health Organization in places where people stay for longer periods of time".'

'Switzerland already has a notable anti-5G lobby, with recent protests against its rollout in Bern, Zurich and Geneva. The Swiss Medical Association has advised caution on 5G, arguing that the most stringent legal principles should be applied because of unanswered questions about the technology's potential to cause damage to the nervous system, or even cancers. Five "popular initiatives" — proposals for legally binding referendums on 5G use — are already in motion in Switzerland. Two have already been formalised and are in the process of collecting the 100,000 signatures needed to trigger nationwide votes that if successful will amend Switzerland's constitution. One will make telecoms companies legally liable for claims of bodily damage caused by radiation from masts unless they can prove otherwise. The other proposes strict and stringent limits on radiation emissions from masts and will give local residents veto power over all new constructions in their area.'

Brian Stein's Diary March 2020

Along comes the coronavirus! At the same time, the development of the 5G roll-out and the realisation by some of the population that this is different from what has gone before and the extent of masts required has caused consternation.

Anti-5G organisations have been springing up across the globe and many scientists have been speaking out about the fact that 5G could be extremely dangerous. This has started to resonate with people in the UK and people are wanting to know why it has not been tested before roll-out. Good question.

Because of the vacuum created by the media in the UK, the government has not had to explain why it is considered to be safe with no research, and being rolled out. This vacuum, together with the acceleration of Covid 19, has created fear and hostility.

Brian Stein's Diary, 5 April 2020

Baseless theories linking the roll-out of 5G with the Covid 19 pandemic began to spread on social media in February. One press report says, 'Oliver Dowden, the Culture Secretary, will confront social media companies this week over the need to curb the spread of the theory.'

Other reports say: 'David Icke has claimed that microwaves would blanket the planet with ultra-high microwave frequencies and that Russia today highlighted the possible dangers of the technology.'

The BBC and news media are conflating 5G causing Covid 19 with legitimate concerns about the roll-out of 5G, thereby labelling anyone concerned about 5G as a conspiracy theorist.

Stopping the roll-out until independent tests are carried out, and peer-reviewed research suggesting 2G/3G/4G and 5G damage the immune system, and thereby cause the worsening of symptoms in some people, are legitimate concerns.

Brian Stein's Diary 8 April 2020

Carol Midgley in The Times writes: 'I am writing this in my silver-lined 5G-resistant knickers – and you?'

'As you know, several 5G masts have been set on fire... as the lockdown causes an outbreak of cretinousness... 5G is suppressing your immune system and doubtless cooking your goolies like two braised chicken nuggets.'

'An Ofcom report in February found that there were no risks from 5G signals and that radiation emitted by tower sites was just 0.039% of recommended exposure limits. Which is why I am writing this wearing my silver-lined 5G-resistant knickers.'

Obviously fully up to date with the latest research for her article. Who is the cretin?

Brian Stein's Diary 12 April 2020

With the rising fear of 5G, and the linking of 5G with coronavirus, the authorities have moved into overdrive. Not only is 5G not associated with causing coronavirus (probable), there is 'no' evidence of harm from 2G/3G/4G or 5G, which is a blatant distortion of the truth.

The BBC seem to have been enlisted to spread the message, and some of the BBC programmes on 5G have been serious distortions of the truth. The 'File on 4' programme was so biased, if it had been anyone other than the BBC I would have found it amusing.

The fact that some people are making money out of people's fears does not mean that ES doesn't exist and microwaves don't harm your health. In the same way, people marketing fake cures for cancer doesn't mean cancer does not exist. It simply means that people will take advantage of people's fears.

The more evidence being produced that EMFs are harmful to our health, the louder the authorities are shouting that it is completely safe.

I think the authorities are starting to believe the lies they spread.

Brian Stein's Diary, 19 April 2020

'*5G causes headaches, but mainly for gullible celebrities*' *(Sunday Times April 19th).*

'*The new mobile networks have no links to Covid-19 or cancer*'.

The Times is conflating the two issues. Most of the peer-reviewed independent research is clearly showing a link between microwaves and cancer. The article continues to link Covid-19 scare stories with legitimate concerns, in a serious attempt to prove the safety of microwaves when the research says the opposite. The BBC and press regularly dismiss peer-reviewed research in favour of spin.

The article continues: '*David Robert Grimes, a physicist and cancer researcher, quotes the reason for these renewed concerns as a piece in Scientific American in October by a public health researcher called Joel Moskowitz, entitled:* '*We Have No Reason to Believe 5G is Safe.*' *It attracted significant attention.*'

'*Moskowitz's piece relied on a small study* (the largest ever undertaken) *looking at cancer incidences in rats, which found that 2G (not 5G)* (but still microwaves below the ICNIRP guidelines) *radio waves were associated with higher rates of some cancers. But he didn't mention that this was only in male rats* (not true, the cancer was more prevalent in male rats, but female rats had pre-cancer cells which the unexposed group did not), *on average the rats that had been exposed to 2G radiation lived longer than the ones that hadn't.*' (Not true, the exposed rats lived 2/3 days longer with cancer than the unexposed rats, which is scientifically irrelevant.) (See Radiation Research Trust website National Toxicology Program study presented by Ron Melnick, who corrects David Robert Grimes' junk science).

Grimes makes spin the headlines, while the top cancer specialists from around the world who classified microwaves as possibly carcinogenic get ignored.

Brian Stein's Diary 25 April 2020

5G masts on lamp posts can raise cash, is the official suggestion. The government has encouraged councils to consider installing 5G masts on lamp posts to fund repair for roads.

Brian Stein's Diary, May/June 2020

Reported in The Times that the Scientific Pandemic Influenza Modelling Committee (SPI-M) which advises 'Sage' on February 10th stated: 'It is a realistic probability that there is already sustained transmission (of coronavirus) in the UK, or it will become established in the coming weeks.'

On the 25th February, Public Health England told the care sector 'the current position in the UK' was that 'there is currently no transmission of Covid-19 in the community.' PHE advised that it remains 'very unlikely that people receiving care in a care home or the community will become infected.' The NHS therefore sent patients into care homes whose occupants were the most endangered.

BBC's 'File on 4' programme on care homes quoted that PHE knew of care home outbreaks before the lockdown and after and didn't reveal the information/problem until end of April.

I think this is relevant to the EMF debate because this is precisely the experience of competence and incompetence that Public Health England has demonstrated to the EMF debate for the last 20 years.

Precisely, not following the science, but being used as a political football by the government in pretending to follow the science, when actually bending the science and making political decisions to benefit the economy.

Brussels, June 2020

Michele Rivasi and Klaus Buchner were members of the European Parliament. They commissioned, co-ordinated and published the report 'The International Commission on Non-Ionizing Radiation Protection: Conflicts of interest, corporate interests and the push for 5G.' In their endeavour, they were inspired and assisted by the journalistic organisation *Investigate Europe*.

This was a publicly-funded landmark study which examined, identified and exposed the conflicts of interest between ICNIRP, the self-styled regulatory body acting in the interests of the consumer, and the mobile phone industry who were to all intents and purposes ICNIRP's paymasters. The report revealed in unprecedented detail the tactics of ICNIRP over three decades and the identities of its key personalities (**See Appendix 9**).

Brian Stein's Diary 18 July 2020

The Minister for Health has called for an urgent review of England's coronavirus death toll, after recognising that everyone who has ever tested positive is included in the deaths, regardless of their cause of death.

The methodology used by Public Health England is called into question by Carl Heneghan from Oxford University and Yoon Loke from East Anglia University, who wrote 'A patient who has tested positive, but been successfully discharged, will still still be counted as a Covid death even if they had a heart attack, or are run over by a bus three months later.'

The ES community has been claiming that Public Health England is incompetent for the last 20 years with regard to new illnesses. It takes Covid to expose them as incompetent to the general public.

Brian Stein's Diary 23 July 2020

England: phone mast planning rules scrapped to improve 5G.

France: mayors band together to halt Macron's 5G network. 'French mayors have called a halt to the construction of 5G mobile masts until health risks have been assessed.'

Ann Vignot, mayor or Besancon, tweeted: '5G causes problems for public health.'

The great divide. One country allowed to talk about the peer-reviewed science, the other has banned the debate about 5G and health and is legislating to allow roll-out without considering the peer-reviewed scientific side effects.

A Tale of Two Cities.

Brian Stein's Diary 23 July 2020

Fertility rate for women under 30 is lowest on record.

Many people will wonder what these diary comments mean. They can easily be disputed. However, when you join the dots, the way society is changing, the experience of the electrically hypersensitive community and the peer-reviewed research, you find convincing evidence that we have a serious problem with microwaves significantly below the ICNIRP and Public Health England guidelines. Join the... dots... and... follow... the money. £.

*

The National Toxicology Program, the Ramazzini Institute findings, the London Conference, the Phonegate lawsuit in California, the Turin Court ruling , the Swiss Government and the European Parliament were the latest to show that existing wireless radiation safety standards were dangerous to human health whether you were online or not. 5G, in inadequately-regulated form, would increase this danger to an unprecedented degree and on an unprecedented scale.

This had already been demonstrated for many years by millions of animals and creatures in the wild, and in the laboratory, where they had proved the disruptive and carcinogenic effects of non-thermal microwave radiation on bioactivity.

Until the multi-trillion dollar mobile industry and ICNIRP acknowledged that they were wrong, and the worldwide community of independent peer-reviewed scientists were right, hundreds of thousands of mice and rats would go on being sacrificed in the cause of exposing the microwave delusion.

9 The Birds and the Bees (and the Rats and the Bats)

'For decades, research results have been freely accessible which show that the natural electric and magnetic fields and its variations are vital conditions for the orientation and navigation of a whole range of animals. Likewise, for many decades it has also been well known in science that we humans depend on these natural factors for numerous vital functions.'

'Today, however, this natural information and function system of humans, animals and plants becomes superimposed by a never before existing density and intensity of artificial magnetic, electric and electromagnetic fields of numerous mobile and communication radio technologies. The consequences repeatedly predicted over many decades by the critics of this development should now no longer be overlooked. Bees and other insects disappear, birds avoid certain places and are disorientated in other places. Man suffers from malfunctions and diseases; and as these become hereditary, passes them on as damages to the next generation.'

– Dr Ulrich Warnke, University of Saarland, Germany

While the war of words, of rigorously-gathered scientific evidence and industry-funded counter-propaganda, went on between humans, it was a fact that the effects of wireless radiation on animal species aroused concern for their welfare in humans, even as the latter were being induced to believe that wireless radiation was safe.

Unlike humans, animals and insects couldn't speak or sue, take out insurance, or commission studies that proved the psychological theory of electrosensitivity over the physiological theory of electrosensitivity, or the physiological theory of electrosensitivity over the pysychological theory of electrosensitivity: but nor could they lie. And unlike humans, surrounded by microwaves in their homes and offices and classrooms, animals and insects could and did vary their migration patterns; albeit, as the emerging evidence suggested, not always successfully.

Back in 2000, Dr Gerard Hyland had suggested that when it came to microwave masts, pine trees could not pretend, plants did not dissimulate and cows did not imagine things, and he had been punished for it. The number of masts across Britain had multiplied to over 50,000 since then and would go on rising. Yet the alert tones that might have accompanied them were not there.

In 1956, with the Cold War escalating with East Germany and the Soviet Union, a military radar engineer working on the Sussex Downs had witnessed at first hand the effect of 3GHz microwave radiation on migrating birds. The birds – mainly swifts and house martins - would normally gather at between 3,000 and 10,000 feet and spend up to 20 minutes circling chosen landmarks, and then disperse for their foreign destinations. The phenomenon was well-known and documented among personnel at coastal radar stations.

One day, the engineer was testing a new form of radar, with a very fast rise time and short pulse. Suddenly, he noticed that the echoes from the flock of birds had disappeared from the radar. Some time later, reports began to come in to the station of thousands of dead and dying birds spread over a wide area.

The bird deaths reportedly ceased when the frequencies and pulse widths in question ceased to be used. In the late 1980s and early 1990s, Simon Best and Cyril Smith published research warning the government, radio engineers and the public of possible biological damage if similar frequencies and bandwidths were used for wide scale civilian communications. These warnings were reportedly overruled by senior members of the NRPB – later part of the UK Health Protection Agency.

The frequencies and bandwidths in question, meanwhile, were adopted by the mobile phone industry and are in use today.

*

Migratory birds are known to use the earth's geomagnetic field as a source of compass information. There are two competing hypotheses for the primary process underlying the avian magnetic compass: one involves magnetite, the other a magnetically sensitive, chemical reaction.

American and German scientists have shown that oscillating magnetic fields disrupt the magnetic orientation behaviour of migratory birds. The researchers found that robins were disoriented when exposed to a vertically aligned, broadband (0.1-10 MHz) or a single-frequency (7-MHz) field in addition to the geomagnetic field. In the 7-MHz oscillating field, this effect depended on the angle between the oscillating and the geomagnetic fields. The birds exhibited seasonally appropriate, migratory orientation when the oscillating field was parallel to the geomagnetic field, but were disoriented when it was presented at a 24- or 48-degree angle.

In the words of the authors:

'The magnetic compass of birds is light-dependent and exhibits strong lateralization with input coming primarily from the right eye. However, the primary biophysical process underlying this compass remains unexplained. Magnetite, as well as biochemical radical-pair reactions have been hypothesized to mediate sensitivity to Earth-strength, magnetic fields through fundamentally different physical mechanisms.'

So could 50,000 microwave masts, using frequencies and bandwidths similar to those that had killed thousands of birds over the coastal station nearly sixty years earlier, overwhelm even the birds' legendary adaptability? Medium and short wave frequencies had been used since the 1930s with little evidence of any effect on bird behaviour. But stories were beginning to emerge suggesting that research was urgently needed.

In the seaside town of Worthing, the bird population was well cared for by the human one, which accommodated them in hedges, nesting boxes and chimney blocks and fed them in winter. Then, in February 2004, around the local football ground, a fourth TETRA mast went live.

During the same year, the small birds disappeared, leaving the nests empty and the gardens silent. Pigeons and seagulls passed through, but did not roost. Similar phenomena were reported elsewhere.

Only when the mast, which had been illegally installed, was removed, well out of season, did the birds return.

Dr Ulrich Warnke was a lecturer at the University of Saarland, in Germany. Dr Warnke had been researching the effects of man-made electromagnetic fields on wildlife for more than 30 years. At the 2008 Radiation Research Trust conference at the Royal Society in London, he told the audience that 'An unprecedented dense mesh of artificial magnetic, electrical and electromagnetic fields' had been generated, overwhelming the 'natural system of information' on which the species relied. In his opinion, mobile phones, Wi-Fi, electric power lines and similar sources of 'electrosmog' were disrupting nature on a massive scale, causing birds and bees to lose their bearings, fail to reproduce and die.

Dr Warnke believed this could have been responsible for the disappearance of bees in Europe and America in what was known as colony collapse disorder, for the decline of the house sparrow, whose numbers had fallen by half in Britain over the past 30 years, and that it could interfere with bird migration.

The world's natural electrical and magnetic fields, he went on, have had a 'decisive hand in the evolution of species'. Over millions of years, they had learned to use them to work out where they were, the time of day, and the approach of bad weather.

Now, 'man-made technology has created transmitters which have fundamentally changed the natural electromagnetic energies and forces on the earth's surface. Animals that depend on natural electrical, magnetic and electromagnetic fields for their orientation and navigation are confused by the much stronger and constantly changing artificial fields.'

Dr Warnke's research showed that bees exposed to the kinds of electrical fields generated by power lines killed each other and their young, while ones exposed to signals in the same range as mobile 'phones lost much of their homing ability. He cited studies at the University of Koblenz-Landau, where bees failed to return to their hives when digital cordless phones were placed in them. He cited an Austrian survey which noted that two-thirds of beekeepers with mobile phone masts within 300 metres had suffered unexplained colony collapse; and Spanish and Belgian studies showing that the number of sparrows near mobile phone masts fell as radiation increased. Migrating birds, flying in formation, had been seen to split up when approaching the masts.

The Mobile Operators Association, representing Britain's mobile phone companies, countered that an American research group had found collapsing bee colonies in areas with no mobile phone service; while Denis Summers-Smith, 'a leading expert on sparrows', described the link as 'nonsense'. However, a more systematic collation of reports and research relating to links with pulsed microwave radiation revealed growing concern for the wellbeing of the planet's birds.

In America, the U.S. Fish & Wildlife Service voiced its concern in *Potential Radiation Impacts of Cellular Communication Towers on Migratory Birds and Communication Towers on Migratory Birds and Other Wildlife'*. Similar concerns were voiced in India, and now in Britain:

Resonance effects indicate a radical-pair mechanism for avian magnetic compass, (Nature, May 2004)

On the use of magnets to disrupt the physiological compass of birds, (Physical Biology, 2006)

Research on the radical-pair theory of magnetic sensitivity; 'weak electromagnetic fields at appropriate frequencies in the radio frequency (RF) range should disrupt or change magnetic orientation behavior if the magnetic compass were based on radical pair reactions.'

A Model for Photoreceptor-Based Magnetoreception in Birds, (Biophysics Journal, 2000)

Mobile Phones and Vanishing Birds (Institute of Science in Society)

A Possible Effect of Electromagnetic Radiation from Mobile Phone Base Stations on the Number of Breeding House Sparrows (Passer domesticus), Joris Everaert, Dirk Bauwens (*Electromagnetic Biology and Medicine*, Volume 26, Issue 1, January 2007)

The Urban Decline of the House Sparrow (Passer domesticus): A Possible Link with Electromagnetic Radiation, Alfonso Balmori, Örjan Hallberg (*Electromagnetic Biology and Medicine*, Volume 26, Issue 2, April 2007)

Possible Effects of Electromagnetic Fields from Phone Masts on a Population of White Stork (Ciconia ciconia), Alfonso Balmori

The common theme running through these independent research papers was that birds suffered from the effects of exposure to microwave radiation from masts, Wi-Fi routers, DECT and mobile phones. Many more anecdotal reports detailed the disappearance of songbirds following the installation and activation of a mast - and their return after the mast's removal.

*

Dr Warnke and others noted these patterns and the apparent rise in coincidences between microwave radiation events and changes in animal and insect behaviour. In 2008, there was a sudden and apparently inexplicable bee colony collapse across Britain and mainland Europe. Bees were regarded as a barometer of humanity's wellbeing. The Berlin-based Kompetenzinitiative was a coalition of scientists and physicians specialising in research into the environmental effects of electromagnetic fields. Its Scientific

Editor, Professor Dr Karl Richter, wrote to bee associations and beekeepers:

'*Varroa Mite or Electromagnetic Fields?*'

'*New Research into the Death of Bees*'

'*Letter to Beekeepers and Beekeeper Associations*'

'*Dear Board Members and Directors of Beekeeper Associations,*'

'*Dear Beekeepers!*'

'*The death of bees has for some time concerned beekeepers, the media, but also worried scientists who have affiliated themselves with our Kompetenz initiative for the protection of man, environment and democracy (www.kompetenzinitiative.de).*'

'*The disturbing phenomenon is presently predominantly attributed to the Varroa mite in newspapers and periodicals. It remains uncontested that there are such connections. Yet plausible arguments have been put forward explaining that the mite attack also occurs as a result of previous damage to the bees' immune system due to electromagnetic fields.*'

The letter quoted from the findings of Dr. Warnke:

'*Other causes are also discussed, which aim to explain the disappearance of the bees: Single-crop farming, pesticides, the Varroa mite, mobile apiaries, corroded seeds, too severe winters, genetically modified plants. It remains uncontested that these also cause problems. Yet, the fact that for the last two to three years bee death has appeared rather suddenly and spread across countries, can be explained convincingly by none of the above mentioned causes. If the bees simply became excessively weakened and ill, they would have to perish in or in front of the beehive. Yet, in the case of this particular phenomenon, no sick bees are to be found.*'

The letter also cited the existence of HAARP (High-frequency Active Auroral Research Project), operated by the U.S. Air Force and the U.S. Navy near the city of Gakona in Alaska. HAARP consisted of an antenna complex of 180 towers in an uninhabited area, operating on a frequency of 2.5 – 10 MHz. With an output of over 3 million Watts, HAARP was and is the earth's most powerful high frequency radio wave transmitter.

Links were suggested between HAARP and the Colony Collapse Disorder that afflicted bees in Canada, America and in Europe. In 2006, the transmitting power was increased from 960,000 watts to 3.6 million Watts, exactly the same year that an unprecedented disruption in the homing ability of bees was reported across all the areas covered by the transmission.

As Dennis van Engelsdorp of the American Association of Professional Apiculturists at the University of Pennsylvania reported: 'We never saw so many different viruses all at once. Moreover, we have found fungus, flagellate and other microorganisms. This variety of pathogens is confusing.'

Van Engelsdorp noted that the excretory organs of the bees had been attacked, and concluded that some kind of immunodeficiency lay beneath the mysterious phenomena. However, he added: 'Are these pathogens the causal stress factor or the consequence of an entirely different effect?'

It was 'extremely alarming', said Diana Cox-Foster, a member of the Colony Collapse Disorder Working Group, that the deaths were combined with symptoms, 'which until now were never described like that'. The immune system of the animals seemed to have collapsed, with many bees suffering from five to six infections simultaneously.

As the Kompetenzinitiative document went on to describe, bees and other insects, like birds, used the earth's magnetic field and high frequency electromagnetic energy, such as light. They achieve orientation and navigation by means of what are known as free radicals, as well as a simultaneously reacting magnetite conglomerate. Recent, large-scale man-made electromagnetic oscillations in the MHz-range and magnetic impulses in the low frequency range, persistently disturbed the natural orientation and navigation mechanisms created by millions of years of evolution.

Dr Warnke pointed to the physiological makeup of bees and their orientation to the magnetic and electromagnetic field of the earth, and the disruption of the bees' NO (nitric oxide) systems, whereby their management of free radicals would also be disturbed.

'A disturbed Nitric Oxide (NO) system damages learning ability, scent orientation and immune system', he wrote of the central mechanism of action, which was equally applicable to humans.

'If the bees' NO-system is disturbed through the influence of technical magnetic fields, a case also observed in humans, they can no longer orient themselves through scent memory, and their all important learning process necessary for life no longer functions. However, as NO controls the immune system to a large extent, a disturbed NO balance will always affect the organism's immune defense.'

'A case also observed in humans...'

In Britain, Heather Whitney had been the third-year undergraduate who co-authored the paper with Professor Goldsworthy on the biological effects of conditioned water, which had led to his explanation of the mechanism of the biological effects of mobile phones, the cessation of his research students and effective closure of his laboratory facilities at Imperial College, London.

By 2013, Dr Heather Whitney was an award-winning plant scientist at the School of Biological Sciences at the University of Bristol. With her colleagues Dominic Clarke, Gregory Sutton and Daniel Robert, she had published a new study entitled 'Detection and Learning of Floral Electric Fields by Bumblebees'.

The abstract is reproduced here in full:

'Insects use several senses to forage, detecting floral cues such as color, shape, pattern, and volatiles. We report a formerly unappreciated sensory modality in bumblebees (Bombus terrestris), detection of floral electric fields. These fields act as floral cues, which are affected by the visit of naturally charged bees. Like visual cues, floral electric fields exhibit variations in pattern and

structure, which can be discriminated by bumblebees. We also show that such electric field information contributes to the complex array of floral cues that together improve a pollinator's memory of floral rewards. Because floral electric fields can change within seconds, this sensory modality may facilitate rapid and dynamic communication between flowers and their pollinators.'

The *'formerly unappreciated sensory modality'* and *'rapid and dynamic communication'* identified by Dr Whitney and her colleagues were not only a significant scientific advance *per se*, but an encapsulation, literally in microcosm, of the extent to which natural world in all its manifestations thrives and fails to thrive according to the status of electric fields. To discover that such a balance should be even more delicate and beautiful than was previously known was one of the great rewards of science, as both Professor Olle Johansson in Stockholm and Professor Andrew Goldsworthy in London were quick to agree. Furthermore, as Professor Johansson observed, this was 'yet another species ready for the psychiatrists and their cognitive behavioural therapy'.

*

In the risks to the animal species, lay the risks to humans. All around the world, thousands of laboratory rats had involuntarily helped advance the cause of science and a greater understanding of the physiological effects of radiofrequency radiation and electromagnetic fields. Dr Allen Frey in America; Professor Leif Salford in Stockholm; Dr Henry Lai and Narendra P. Singh in America; Dr Jerry Phillips in America; Professor Dariusz Leszczynski in Finland; Professor Lukas Margaritis in Athens; all their rats had been sacrificed after showing the physiological effects on their blood brain barrier, testes, reproductive capability and DNA of exposure to radiofrequency radiation.

If it was one of the many ironies of the battleground of electromagnetic fields that the species closest to humans was the weapon of choice of both sides, the further irony might yet prove to be the rats' revenge on humans: for in the end 'We (i.e not the rats) are the experiment,' as Dr Gerard Hyland put it. Wi-Fi is 'The largest biological experiment ever,' according Professor Leif Salford.

The experiments on captive laboratory animals were accompanied by further field studies into the effects of radiation on wild species. In Britain, where bats were a protected species, the Bat Conservation Trust paper *'The potential impact of radio frequencies and microwaves on wildlife'* described how Wi-Fi antennae transmitted and received radio waves in frequency bands near 2.5 and 4 gigahertz, and how mobile telecommunication systems transmitted at a similar frequency using digitally pulsed signals. Studies into the effect of electromagnetic radiation on foraging bats suggested that bat activity could be reduced when an area free from electromagnetic fields was subjected to electromagnetic fields, but the finding were inconclusive and more research was called for.

Meanwhile, the Bat Conservation Trust advocated a bat equivalent of the Precautionary Principle: the erection of masts should be as far from known roosting locations and flight paths as possible; bat populations within buildings on which masts were installed should be monitored on an annual basis.

In India, the Ministry of Environment and Forests also commissioned studies into the effects on bats of microwave radiation.

In Spain, research scientist Alfonso Balmori had been examining the effects of mobile phone mast radiation on common frog (Rana temporaria) tadpoles.

'An experiment has been made exposing eggs and tadpoles of the common frog (Rana temporaria) to electromagnetic radiation from several mobile (cell) phone antennae located at a distance of 140 meters. The experiment lasted two months, from the egg phase until an advanced phase of tadpole prior to metamorphosis. Measurements of electric field intensity (radiofrequencies and microwaves) in V/m obtained with three different devices were 1.8

to 3.5 V/m. *In the exposed group (n = 70), low coordination of movements, an asynchronous growth, resulting in both big and small tadpoles, and a high mortality (90%) was observed. Regarding the control group (n = 70) under the same conditions but inside a Faraday cage, the coordination of movements was normal, the development was synchronous, and a mortality of 4.2% was obtained. These results indicate that radiation emitted by phone 'masts in a real situation may affect the development and may cause an increase in mortality of exposed tadpoles. This research may have huge implications for the natural world, which is now exposed to high microwave radiation levels from a multitude of 'phone masts.'*

*

Birds, bees; rats, bats; flowers and tadpoles. If the reactions in these species were to be believed, the implications were cataclysmic for animals and insects and for the human genome.

At the conclusion of their research paper (**see link in Appendix 4**), Blake Levitt and Dr Henry Lai stated:

'The increasing popularity of wireless technologies makes understanding actual environmental exposures more critical with each passing day. This also includes any potential effects on wildlife. There is a new environmental concept taking form – that of 'air as habitat' (Manville 2007) for species such as birds, bats and insects in the same way that water is considered habitat for marine life. Until now, air has been considered something 'used' but not necessarily 'lived in' or critical to the survival of species. However, when air is considered habitat, RFR is among the potential pollutants with an ability to adversely affect other species. It is a new area of enquiry deserving of immediate funding and research.'

The industry and parts of the media first ignored, then ridiculed, then threatened the likes of Gerard Hyland and Gerd Oberfeld; the likes of Ulrich Warnke and Cindy Sage; for 'not being scientists' or for carrying out 'pseudoscience'. The inaccuracy of these allegations aside, if these people were so harmless, why were some scientists so hostile to their findings?

As Carl Sagan famously observed: 'Absence of evidence is not evidence of absence.' Now the presence of evidence was mounting. If the pine tree couldn't lie, if the birds and the bees were to be believed, and the rats and the bats, and the tadpoles, and the Danish schoolgirls' watercress, the natural world was under assault from some kind of human activity.

To recognise the risk to animal species is to recognise the risk to ourselves, our children and our children's children.

10 One of Us

'The truth is slow, but it is inexorable.'

– Booker Prize Winner, Richard Flanagan

'First they ignore you, then they ridicule you, then they fight you, then you win'

– Mahatma Gandhi

Brian Stein

Can you imagine living in a city in a flat with neighbours above, below and around you, using Wi-Fi, mobiles and smart meters, and you know you are being made ill by this technology?

Being ES is a devastating condition.

Not only are you being made ill, but the authorities, having admitted that some people will be more sensitive to this technology, are trying to damage your credibility by insisting that although you are being made ill, and there are thousands of scientific papers explaining why you are being made ill, it is nothing to do with microwaves and your illness is psychosomatic.

So not only are you ill, but your friends and family are being convinced that you are suffering from some imaginary fear, and doubting your logic.

I know hundreds of ES sufferers. The vast majority are trying to survive in their environment without moving house. Most are desperate to continue using this technology, and damage themselves further in the process. They were certainly not fearful of the technology: if they had been, they would not now be ES.

Yet scientists with no serious research pontificate that ES people are delusional and simply belong to a section of the community that has always wanted to be hermits. You become reclusive and anti-social because going to friends' houses where they have Wi-Fi, television, smart meters and cordless phones transmitting 24-7, your system is unable to cope.

Transport is difficult. Holidays are difficult. Education is difficult. Shopping is difficult. Going into hospital is difficult.

You have no human rights.

There are millions of severely ES people around the world and hundreds of millions of people who will be mildly sensitive, who are being made ill and have no understanding as to why.

People who suffer from ME will have their condition made worse by EMFs. I believe the vast majority of ME sufferers are actually electrically or chemically sensitive. Many of the people who die from 'sudden death syndrome' will be ES. Their hearts are ES.

Our 'authorities' claim that they are taking 'a precautionary approach' with this technology by suggesting children should limit their use of it – at the same time they are installing Wi-Fi in schools.

I cannot think of anything we are doing in the UK that is 'precautionary'.

Sir William Stewart was the only person in the Health Protection Agency who called for caution and precaution. He appeared on 'Panorama' and suggested we should not install Wi-Fi in schools. Shortly afterwards he was removed from office. Since his removal, the new body, Public Health England, talks of a precautionary approach while doing the opposite.

My advice for ES people:

1. *Do not use a mobile phone.*
2. *Do not live near a mast.*
3. *Try to live in a house that is separate from your neighbours.*
4. *Turn off the electricity at night when you are feeling your worst, or rewire the house so this you can isolate the electricity in your bedroom.*

5   Remove all wireless devices.
6   Limit your use of wired computers.
7   Use a speakerphone.
8   Use an old diesel car.
9   Use a cheap meter to check emission levels.
10 Take a precautionary approach for your children.

There are now over forty studies showing adverse health effects even from very low level emissions from Wi-Fi. The latest studies from Sweden, France and Germany indicate a 400% increase in cancer in mice kept in a Wi-Fi environment.

The response from ICNRP and the UK Health Protection Agency is similar to that of the Russian authorities denying there is anything to answer when a 300 page dossier details a regime of cheating in athletics. There is no credible evidence – the evidence is groundless. While thousands of peer-reviewed papers show the damaging effects of EMFs, Wi-Fi, mobile 'phones and 'smart' meters, the authorities maintain there is no credible evidence. When an authority has no credible response, it hopes the accusations will go away if a denial is issued by high level officials who couldn't possibly be involved in duplicity.

The British authorities did this with cigarettes and asbestos, Hillsborough and Jimmy Saville. In these cases, we did not learn the lessons of the past, we made the situation worse before denial became fruitless and the evidence obvious. In order for this to happen, however, the media has to confront the truth – and this is difficult when 50% of all media spend comes from the wireless industry.

The conspiracy is one of self-interest. Which newspaper is going to accuse their main advertiser that they are involved in the biggest cover up in the history of modern business and health?

*

In 1932, the German doctor Erwin Schliephake published scientific data in a German medical weekly about radio *transmitter-induced 'microwave' or 'radio wave' sickness with the following symptoms: severe tiredness and fatigue during the day, fitful sleep in the night, headaches to the point of intolerability and high susceptibility to infection – exactly the same as electrically-sensitive people are suffering over 80 years later.*

Wireless devices cause cancer. There is strong evidence of pre-natal exposure harming the foetus. Adverse effects can include cardiac symptoms and compromised brain function and cognitive ability. Low levels of radio frequency radiation (Wi-Fi and mobile phones) can compromise the blood-brain barrier and damage the brain (Salford, Persson). This can increase the risk of neurodegenerative conditions including Parkinson's Disease.

Cognitive impairment from Wi-Fi has been shown by Professors Kundi and Moesgeller of Vienna Medical University.

Meanwhile, academics debate the concentration issues of students and recommend mobile devices are not used in schools because they possibly interfere with learning: all without referring to research showing brain damage and adverse effects on neurotransmitters (Moesgeller, Scheiner, Lai, Hareuveny, Meiran, Morgalist, Cherry, Luria, Elyahu).

If the electrically-sensitive community proves its condition, Disability Discrimination legislation will cause the community many inconveniences. The right of individuals not to be irradiated will cause lovers of this technology serious inconvenices as opposed to the ES community suffering serious health issues. The answer is therefore to deny the possibility and the philosophy of the greatest good for the majority.

Can you imagine this being allowed to happen for people in wheelchairs, the deaf, the blind?

When challenging the Chair of the Smart Meter roll-out, who agreed to meet me and then reneged on the meeting, she 'explained' that if I had the right not to have a smart meter, then it was only right that other people should have the right to have a smart meter. When I asked if people who were ES refused a smart meter, what would happen when the person in the flat above and below installed one, and how that right not to be irradiated would work, she refused to answer.

*

Can you imagine a piece of Wi-Fi research indicating a significant increase in cancer at a time when all our schools are installing routers? It should generate interest from the Health Protection Agency and the media – but no. One piece of research – no interest.

Now imagine the research being replicated and finding the same results. Surely interest from the Health Protection Agency and the media? But no. The research is 'flawed' – no interest.

Now imagine a government scientist, sceptical of the results, replicating the research, correcting the supposed 'flaws', and finding exactly the same results – a 400% increase in cancers in mice kept in a Wi-Fi environment. Surely interest, concern, from the Health Protection Agency and the media? But no.

Instead, an even 'better' response – ignore it. That way it doesn't exist. No debate.

This is the UK response to repeated Wi-Fi research showing significant increases in cancers. The authorities have found that simply ignoring any research by the health profession and the press is the 'best' response. No debate.

There are now over 40 research papers showing the serious ill-effects of Wi-Fi. Other research shows that smartphones and tablets emit the kind of light that disrupts the human body clock:

'For a good night's sleep, stop taking the tablets' – The Times, 17.11.2015.

As an ES person I can assure you that smartphones and tablets disrupt sleep – but the emission of light is minor compared with the emission of EMFs, and the volume of research showing this is considerably more than that showing the effects of the emission of light. However, it is not 'politically correct' to blame EMFs.

In 2009, evidence was supplied of cognitive impairment from Wi-Fi by Professors Kundi and Mosgoeller of Vienna Medical University. Brain wave changes continued long after exposure. Since then, numerous reports have been published showing:

'Smartphones Make Us Dumb' – The Times, 11.10.2015

Professor Turkle of the Faculty of Social Sciences at Massachusetts Institute of Technology (MIT) warned that family conversation is being destroyed and such 'phones 'need a health warning' – The Times, 12.10.2015

The Strategic Society Centre warned that 'There is enough evidence for policy makers and companies to be worried about the effects these technologies and social media are having on some children.'

'Want to be happier? Give up Facebook.' – The Times 11.11.2015'

'Giving up Facebook boosts happiness and reduces anger – Social media damages the mental health of young people' – Researchers at the Happiness Institute in Copenhagen.

'Zapping brains can reduce faith in God, claims a researcher at the University of California and York' – The Times 15.10.2015'

Amid all this research showing the way our young people's brains are being changed by social media, there is no mention of the research showing the way EMFs actually alter the brain. The assumption made is that it is the social interaction that is causing these changes and it is nothing to do with the way EMFs alter brain function.

'Pigeon's inner magnetism could help us find the way' – The Times 17.11.2015'

Scientists at Beijing University have found a protein bundle buried in the cells of pigeons, fruit flies and monarch butterflies that binds to iron atoms and uses them to snap navigation molecules to face north.

Scientists have also discovered magnetic proteins in the retinal nerves of animals, which allow them to navigate using the Earth's magnetic field. It is unlikely that this magnetic field is not disrupted by man-made EMFs – contributing to the disappearance of birds, bees, insects and fish who survive by the use of these protein bundles to find their way home and to breeding grounds.

Researchers have also discovered that humans express these same proteins, raising the prospect that we too have some ability to sense the magnetic field.

*

Galileo was convicted by the Inquisition and placed under house arrest for revealing the Earth was not the centre of the universe - the standard delusional paradigm at the time.

In today's economy, the delusion is that microwaves below the ICNIRP guidelines are safe, and any scientist who disputes this paradigm is accused of scientific fraud, unreliability, activism - the equivalent of accusing a teacher of child abuse – and destroying the scientist's credibility.

*

The Equality Act defines a disabled person as one who has a physical or mental impairment that has a substantial and long-term adverse effect on his or her ability to carry out normal everyday activities.

An ES person is unable to carry out some of the most basic acts of our society. They are unable to work, shop or visit in a Wi-Fi environment, watch TV, use a computer, go on holiday. All these activities fit into the above description, but would require a massive change in our society to allow these people to live a normal life. It is easier therefore to deny its existence and assert that people who are troubled by EMFs are imagining it.

*

In the field of fertility research, over 80% of studies show the adverse effects of wireless signals on male fertility. ICNIRP and Public Health England have regularly stated that 'there is no evidence of ill-health and microwave exposure below the ICNIRP guidelines.'

As more and more evidence to the contrary has been produced, they have changed their stance to 'there is no <u>consistent</u> evidence of ill-health and microwave exposure below the ICNIRP guidelines.'

As more and more consistent, repeated evidence has been produced, they have changed their stance to 'there is no <u>consistent, reliable</u> evidence of ill-health and microwave exposure below the ICNIRP guidelines.'

When challenged as to what they mean by 'reliable', they explain that they 'weight' the evidence by its reliability. The definition of this 'reliability' is according to ICNIRP's definition of science where science suits their position.

Thus, the 'evidence' to support their assertion that it is safe is weighted more heavily than the evidence they believe is 'unreliable' – and hence there is 'no evidence' of microwaves below the ICNIRP guidelines being consistently unsafe.

*

Recent research into Wi-Fi has consistently shown that mice exposed to it have a 200-400% increase in cancer. Recent research with rabbits has shown that Wi-Fi exposure affects their heart rhythm, blood pressure and cardiovascular system.

In the UK, we install Wi-Fi in our schools and hospitals, and the 'smart' meter system introduced by the government is a Wi-Fi system.

Because of concerns expressed by some people in the UK, Public Health England have spent half a million pounds conducting tests to 'reassure' the population. These 'tests' consist of checking that the Wi-Fi signals in schools, hospitals and smart meters are below the ICNIRP guidelines – which they are. Everyone therefore can be 'reassured' that they are safe.

*However, the recent research showing alarming health problems from Wi-Fi exposure has all been conducted at levels significantly **below** the ICNIRP guidelines – Public Health England's assurances are therefore meaningless.*

*

Whenever ES people are checked for psychological problems, they are generally found to be normal. The 'nocebo' hypothesis attributed to people 'thinking' they are ES has been shown to be false on numerous occasions.

The idea that people become fearful of EMFs because they are fearful of technology is preposterous and not based on any serious scientific evaluation. Yet it is perpetuated by much of the British media and the medical profession.

The vast majority of people becoming ES do so because they have embraced the technology and then been damaged by it. They are damaged because they have overused the technology and not because they are fearful of it.

*

Studies show that the removal of mobile phones base stations in other countries significantly improves the health of the surrounding population. In spite of the fact that UK mobile phone base stations use exactly the same frequencies and technology, no such studies have ever taken place on the health of the population surrounding mobile phone base stations in this country.

The ICNIRP guidelines are based on the knowledge of direct acute effects such as electric shock and tissue heating. The guidelines allow the general public to be exposed to one quintillian - 1 to the power 18-fold, or 1,000,000,000,000,000,000 times more electromagnetic fields than the natural background level thirty years ago.

When challenged, ICNIRP state that their guidelines are for acute thermal effects and not for chronic biological effects, which are for each individual country to evaluate and introduce guidelines accordingly. In the UK, the ICNIRP guidelines are accepted as the norm, and no guidelines are deemed necessary for chronic biological effects, which they assert are not 'consistently repeatable.'

There are therefore no guidelines to protect us from the thousands of peer-reviewed scientific papers showing damage to the nervous system, respiratory system, gastrointestinal system, endocrine system, cardiovascular system, dermatological system, genito-urinary system and similar complaints being experienced by ES people.

Around 40% of the world's population - Russia, China, India, Switzerland, Italy, Austria, Luxembourg, Belgium and Lichtenstein - have tighter safety standards than the UK. France has banned the use of Wi-Fi in kindergartens.

*

The European Convention on Human Rights, Article 2:

Right to Life: Breached.

Protection of Children: Breached.

Protection of Embryos/Foetus: Breached.

Protection of Pregnant Women: Breached.

*

Modern living is leading to a 'hidden' epidemic of neurological disease. A study published in the journal 'Surgical Neurology

International' compares 21 western countries between 1989 and 2010 and finds that dementias in adults are starting a decade earlier than they used to.

Professor Colin Pritchard of Bournemouth University led the study: 'The rate of increase in such a short time suggests a silent or even a 'hidden' epidemic in which environmental factors must play a major part.'

All ES people would endorse the fact that being in a Wi-Fi or EMF field causes brain fog, confusion and serious memory problems.

The world's most 'Hi-Tech' country, South Korea, is now reporting adults in their 30s with dementia.

*

In 2015, after Gemany's Alex Lerchl had ridiculed research into Wi-Fi causing cancer, he was asked by the German government to replicate the research using methods he thought might be more acceptable to ascertain the truth.

His studies, a replica of those from Sweden, France and Germany, were published in March 2015. They found that weak mobile phone signals promote the growth of tumours in mice. The signals used radiation levels that did not cause heating and are well below current safety standards.

*

The Council of Europe has called on governments to give more information and run awareness-raising campaigns on the potentially harmful biological effects of electromagnetic fields. When the Radiation Research Trust ran such a campaign in the UK, the Advertising Standards Authority banned it.

What are the symptoms?

Sleep problems.

Anxiety.

Irritability.

Headaches.

Tinnitus.

Concentration and memory problems.

Fatigue.

Disorientation, dizziness and balance problems.

Eye problems.

Cardiac problems.

Cramps.

Body pain.

Nausea, 'flu-like symptoms.

Nose bleeds.

Respiratory problems.

Skin rashes.

Urinary problems.

Thyroid problems.

Diabetes.

High blood pressure.

All these symptoms are exacerbated by being in a microwave environment.

Because these symptoms are so wide-ranging, the UK health authorities feel able to ridicule the concerns of ES people for 'blaming every problem on EMFs.' However, peer-reviewed research shows that EMFs cause these problems.

EMFs also advance the ageing process. All the symptoms above are caused by advancing age, but because of the biological effects of EMFs they are being experienced by much younger age groups.

Each of us has a natural predisposition to suffer from particular illnesses, be it cancer, heart problems or dementia. As a result of living in a Wi-Fi environment, we are accelerating our own natural ageing and suffering from these illnesses in our 30s, 40s and 50s, instead of our 50s, 60s and 70s.

*

Constantly, when confronted with these fears, the UK Health Protection Agency, Public Health England, local councils, mast owners and mobile 'phone companies repeat the mantra that emission levels 'conform with all government and international standards.'

It is only when you question and research the subject that you realise this is simply a falsehood that enables intelligent and highly-educated people to mislead the population.

The truth is, there are no standards.

The standards that exist are simply to prevent thermal, acute health effects. No standards exist to protect us from the low level, chronic effects that thousands of peer-reviewed research papers show cause harmful and damaging consequences. There are no standards to protect us from the biological damage.

This is the microwave delusion.

ICNIRP is an industry-populated committee of belief in thermal effects, so biological effects do not count. Food & Drug Administration is the spokesperson of the USA, Public Health England is the spokesperson of the UK. Each is heavily influenced by their respective governments and their respective governments are indebted to the wireless industry for the economy, taxes and the sale of 2/3/4/5G networks.

They are therefor heavily compromised and influenced by the money at stake. This is a clear conflict of interest.

Cancer Research UK receives significant funding from the mobile phone industry, including Hutchison Whampoa. Cancer Research UK have also sponsored 'Wi-Fi seats' for the 'benefit' of the public on streets around London and the UK.

During the tobacco scandal, the largest donor to the American Cancer Society (ACS) was the tobacco industry. The ACS declared tobacco to be safe and studies showing otherwise to be unconvincing.

Conflicts of interest are usually safeguarded by the three pillars of society – State, Judiciary and the Media. In this instance, there is no proper safeguard.

The State has a conflict of interest. The Media, because of their own digital strategy, for which 50% of advertising revenues comes from the wireless industry, have a conflict of interest. The Judiciary, because of the positioning of the State and the Media, have no interest. At the expense of the common good, the three pillars of society show no appetite for properly safeguarding the public's health from a wireless industry which has set up in business to take maximum advantage of the digital age.

Brian Stein, 2020

AFTERWORD

Elizabeth Barris continued her class action over the damage to health caused by 'smart' meters against Pacific Gas & Electric and Edison in Washington and to campaign for greater transparency from government and industry over EMFs.

Michael Bevington continued as Head of Classics at Stowe School, and compiled a list of peer-reviewed independent research papers on mobile phones and microwave radiation (see **Appendix 1**).

George Carlo the one-time American cell phone industry-funded researcher, continued to liaise with ES campaigners and independent scientists in the UK and around the world. Pressed by Dr Louis Slesin of *Microwave News* twenty years on to produce the WTR papers, Carlo said he was 'travelling in Europe' but would welcome 'an honest exchange' when he got back.

Anne and Bernadette Cautain Touloumonde spent at least three years living away from EMFs in a remote cave in the Vercors range in France.

Professor Lawrie Challis, OBE the British Government advisor and Emeritus Professor of Physics at the University of Nottingham who dismissed fears of health threats from mobile phone base stations, died in 2017.

Frank Clegg, former head of Microsoft in Canada, continued his campaign for a safer electromagnetic environment in Canadian schools.

Devra Davis remained America's most prominent critic of the risks from the cell phone industry's safety standards on unborn babies, pregnant women and human fertility, and continued to lead the Environmental Health Trust.

Dr Allan Frey the American scientist who pioneered research into the effects of non-thermal radiation on the blood-brain barrier, continued in his 80s to work as a scientist at Randomline Inc, Maryland USA. He continued to be consulted by the media as a pioneer of the research into the health hazards of cell phones.

Debra Fry and her husband Charles Newman parents of the late Jenny Fry continued to campaign for the removal of Wi-Fi from nurseries and schools and to secure 'justice for Jenny'.

Professor Andrew Goldsworthy retired from Imperial College, London, and produced the paper in **Appendix 2**.

Professor Yury Grigoriev Russia's leading scientist in the field of radiation continued to speak out about the need of governments and the European Union to acknowledge the health hazards of microwave radiation and electromagnetic fields.

In 2018, he was a contributor to 'Mobile Communications and Public Health' edited by Marko Markov and published in Britain by Taylor and Francis. The book was also distributed in the US.

Sissel Halmoy the former rocket scientist continued to campaign for greater government recognition of the health dangers of microwave radiation and EMFs as Norway chair of the International EMF Alliance.

Professor Lennart Hardell continued his independent research in Sweden into the physiological effects of microwave radiation and electromagnetic fields. He and **Michael Carlberg** published the paper summarised in **Appendix 3**.

Dr Magda Havas continued her researches at Trent University, Ontario.

Professor Denis Henshaw retired as Emeritus Professor at the School of Chemistry, the University of Bristol. He remained active as a consultant concerning the dangers to health of EMFs and non-thermal wireless radiation.

Dr Gerard Hyland the British physicist who raised concerns about the biological effects of mobile phone masts to the British Government in 1999, in the *Lancet* in 2000 and to the European

Parliament in 2001, took early retirement from Warwick University allegedly after 'high level' pressures were brought against his work on the biological effects of electromagnetic fields. He remained an Associate Fellow of Warwick University and became an Executive Member of the International Institute of Biophysics at Neuss-Holzheim in Germany.

He continued to maintain that the safety thresholds regarding masts in the UK were 'wholly inadequate' and that Government and the mobile phone industry enjoyed an unhealthy relationship at the expense of public health and safety: 'We are the experiment,' as he put it.

Phil Inkley lived in a mobile caravan in Hampshire. After 'coming out' in the *Daily Mail* he received an equal measure of sympathy and abuse in the blogosphere – neither of which he could access with any degree of safety. In America his story was taken up by We Are The Evidence (WATE) the wireless technology injured advocacy group.

Professor Olle Johansson continued in post at the Karolinska Institute in Stockholm, Sweden until May, 2016, when he was notified that his services were no longer required on the grounds that he lacked funding, and 'electrohypersensitivity does not exist any longer.' He continued to be active as an independent scientist and researcher into the health dangers of Wi-Fi and EMFs.

Dr Henry Lai and **Blake Levitt** published the paper linked in **Appendix 4.**

Professor Dariusz Leszczynski continued as a research professor at the Radiation and Nuclear Research Authority in Finland, and to speak about the dangers of current industry safety standards for Wi-Fi and EMFs at universities and conferences around the world.

Dr Erica Mallery-Blythe continued to advise electrically-sensitive people, schools and parents and campaign with **Brian Stein** and **Radiation Research Trust (RRT).**

Dr Ron Melnick continued to speak on the conclusions of the National Toxicology Program findings.

Dr Samuel Milham, like **Allan Frey** and **Henry Lai**, remained a frequently-consulted source for his pioneering work regarding the health effects of EMFs and wireless technology under industry-regulated safety thresholds:

Indio, California

What we really need is a film, documentary or coverage by a major TV show. I'm desperate to get the word out, but the media and the government have been corrupted by utility and cell phone money. Since I wrote the book ('Dirty Electricity') I've discovered that smart meters are adding a 50 KHz signal to the grid, earth and air here in California. Again, like photovoltaic solar and wind turbines, the culprit is the switching power supply in each one of them.

Gerd Oberfeld withdrew from the debate surrounding the health effects of EMFs after alleged legal pressure from the mobile industry.

Eileen O'Connor continued to campaign on behalf of the UK Radiation Research Trust for government action on EMFs and microwave radiation safety thresholds in Britain and Brussels.

Professor Martin Pall continued to predicate the effects of safety guideline failure in the roll out of 5G.

Dr Dimitris Panagopoulos continued the research that was among the first to show the damaging effects of microwaves and other man-made EMFs on DNA and reproduction.

Alasdair Philips continued to 'sweep' people's homes and workplaces for Wi-Fi levels and advise on the reduction of electrosmog.

Dr Michael Repacholi continued to defend the position on mobile phone industry safety standards he had held for three decades.

Dr James Rubin continued his researches into the 'psychological' explanations of the health hazards of EMFs and Wi-Fi at King's College, London.

Cindy Sage continued to run Sage Consulting and with others to lead the Bioinitiative project in California.

Professor Leif Salford retired from the Rausing Laboratory in Sweden. His work on EMFs and leakage in the blood-brain barrier was carried on by his former assistant **Henrietta Nittby**.

Dr Diana Samways continued to sweep the homes of friends concerned about the health effects of electromagnetic fields: 'They acknowledge the findings,' she observed, 'but the technology is just too convenient.'

Per Segerback of Ericsson/Elemtel and one of the first 'canaries in the coalmine' was 'let go' by Ericsson in 1999 and moved to a cabin on a remote nature reserve seventy-five miles north-east of Stockholm.

Sweden remained the only country in the world officially to recognise electrosensitivity, a condition from which it acknowledged 250,000 Swedes – 3% of the population – suffered to varying degrees.

Anne Silk continued to research and publish on a range of issues concerning environmental health.

Dr Louis Slesin in New York continued to edit *Microwave News*. ('Meticulously researched and thoroughly documented', *Time* Magazine.)

Brian Stein the subject and co-author of this book retired as Chief Executive of Samworth Brothers, having grown the business from £100 million to nearly £1 billion. His leaving celebrations included a party in the boardroom of Liverpool FC, where he was accorded the rare honour of being allowed to lift the European Cup. He became Chairman of Governors of an Academy in Nottingham City and was awarded Lifetime Achievement Awards by Tesco and the *Leicester Mercury*.

In 2013, he was made a CBE in the Queen's Birthday Honours List for services to business and the community. In 2015, he was invited to discuss the acquisition of land to create the first official

British EMF-free 'white zone' in the Scottish borders. In the same year, he was diagnosed with prostate cancer, which his consultant informed him could have taken up to eight years to develop. It was eight years since he had participated in the Essex Trials. At the time of writing he was in remission.

He is a director of the Nova Education Trust, a multi-academy trust based in Nottinghamshire, UK. In 2019, he chaired the EM-Radiation Research Trust Radiation Health 2019 International Conference in London. Following the success of the conference, EM-Radiation Research Trust decided to become a membership organisation producing regular updates on the public health hazards of 5G.

Sir William Stewart's 'Precautionary Principle' proposed in the 2000 Stewart Report, while generally ignored by the UK Health Protection Agency and Public Health England, remains the benchmark for safety standards in schools in many European countries.

Dr Andrew Tresidder continued to practice as a GP in Somerset.

The Undercover Epidemiologist and colleague continued to send their findings 'up the line'.

Dr Andrea Vornoli continued his research at the Ramazzini Institute into the long-term effects of mobile phone microwave radiation on bioactivity.

Dr Ulrich Warnke continued his research into the health effects of EMFs and microwave radiation on animals and insects at the University of the Saarland. He is now retired.

Thomas E. Wheeler the American cell phone industry lobbyist and former President of CTIA, became a venture capitalist, trustee of the John F. Kennedy Centre and was appointed to President Obama's Intelligence Advisory Board. He resigned on the election of Donald Trump.

Dr Heather Whitney, having studied as a doctoral student under **Professor Andrew Goldsworthy**, continued her research as a plant scientist at the University of Bristol. In 2011, she was awarded the L'Oreal-UNESCO UK and Ireland For Women in Science Fellowship. In 2012, she was awarded the Society for Experimental Biology's President's Medal in Plant Sciences.

CHAPTER NOTES

1: One of Us is Mad

Brian Stein diaries 2005-2020; interviews with Brian Stein, 2012-2020.

2: The Diseases of Civilisation: A Brief History

Beard, G. M., 'Neurasthenia, or nervous exhaustion', *Boston Medical & Surgical Journal*, 80. 1869; John J. O'Neill, 1968; Schliephake E (1932) "Arbeitsgebiete auf dem Kurzwellengebeit" ("Fields in the shortwave region"), *Deutsche Medizinische Wochen-schrift* 32,S. 1235-1240; Daily, L.E., 'A clinical study of the results of exposure of laboratory personnel to radar and high frequency radiation', *US Naval Bulletin*, 41, 1943; Ginzburg, Sadchikova et al., 1968 (Roger Coghill, 1998; "The Invisible Threat: The Stifled Story of Electric Waves," *Saturday Review* 6 (15 September 1979), pp. 16- 20; http://andrewamarino.com/blog/wp-content/uploads/2013/01/SatRev1979.pdf ; http://www.nytimes.com/1986/12/11/obituaries/walter-j-stoessel-jr-dies-at-66-a-former-ambassador-to-moscow.html; Christopher Ketcham 'Warning: High Frequency' Earth *Island Journal*, November, 2012 and 'Warning: Your Cell Phone May Be Bad for Your Health' *GQ* magazine February, 2010; Devra Davis 'Disconnect'; George Carlo and Martin Schram 'Cell Phones: Invisible Hazards in the Wireless Age' Carroll & Graf, NYC, 2001; Gunni Nordstrom 'In a Special Taxi and an Iron-Clad Room' *TCO Newspaper* 18 June, 1993; www.christian-ecology.co.uk; Rigmor Granlund-Lind and John Lind 'Black on White: Voices and Witnesses about Electrohypersensitivity: The Swedish Experience' Mimers Brunn, Sweden 2005; 'Mobile phones and Health' Department of Health, January, 2002; *Dagbladet* 9 March, 2002; *The Engineer*: 30 August-12 September, 2002; Anne Silk paper Prague 25 October,

2004 and interview 9 January, 2013: the *Daily Telegraph*, 24 January, 2005; Mast Action UK Press Release, 24 October, 2005; 'Electrosmog in the Environment' Swiss Agency for the Environment, Forests and Landscape SAEFL, Berne, Switzerland, 2005; *Daily Mail* 20 February, 2007; *Times Online* 15 April, 2007; BBC website 30 November, 2007; Dr Diana Samways paper and interview; interviews with Brian Stein; Radiation Research Trust records; *Romandie News*, 29 October, 2011; *Le Dauphine* 4 December, 2011; *Daily Telegraph* 1 February, 2012; *ES-UK News* March, 2012. Numerous accounts for George Carlo of WTR and Tom Wheeler of CTIA include Mark Hertsgaard and Mark Dowie in *The Nation* 29 March 2018 and *The Observer* 14 July, 2018; Dr Louis Slesin in *Microwave News*, 16 July 2018.

3: Into the Electrostorm

Dr Samuel Milham 'Dirty Electricity', 2010; 'Resonance' James Russell; Carlo and Schram; *Times of India* 7 January, 2012; Professor Girish Kumar report; *ES-UK News* March 2012; *ES-UK News* March 2012; Gye and Park, The Korean Society for Reproductive Medicine 2012; *Aftenbladet* 12 and 13 April, 2013; *Microwave News* 16 November, 2012; *The Sun* 16 November, 2012; Laura Page, the *Guardian* 20 July, 2012; Michael Carlberg and Lennart Hardell, *On the association between glioma, wireless 'phones, heredity and ionising radiation* 6 July, 2012; *Formby Times* 4 September, 2012; Eileen O'Connor and Sissel Halmoy interviews 2013; Radiation Research Trust Press Release September, 2012; Dimitris J. Panogopoulos 'Gametogenesis' paper 2012; Marcolini article, Reuters 19 October, 2012; Marcolini Judge's Conclusion, 12 October, 2012; Didier Bellins, Belgacom and Belgian Royal Decree, Expatica.com 28 February, 2013 and RBTF 25 February, 2013; EU Brussels DG Sanco Unit D3 Risk Assessment EMF Meeting 20130220; http://takebackyourpower.net/emf-on-trial-australia-and-israel-cases-may-be-precedent-setting; http://aaemonline.org/images/LettertoLAUSD.pdf; Le Parisien.fr/AFP, 19 March, 2013; http://www.leparisien.fr/societe/ondes-electromagnetiques-le-principe-de-precaution-bientot-dansles-ecoles-19-03-2013-2653379.php; Joseph Stromberg/*Future Tense*, 12 April 2013; *Blurt Music News* Virginia, 23 January, 2013; *Native News* 13 June, 2013; http://www.scribd.com/doc/146337041/Biological-Effects-From-RF-Radiation-and-Implications-for-Smart-Meters-June 5-2013; 'Mobile Phone Use and the Risk of Skin Cancer: A National Cohort Study in Denmark', *Am J Epidemiol.* 20 June, 2013; http://mastsanity.org/health-52/research/324-experiments-with-cress-in-the-9th-grade-attracts-international-attention-denmark-16th May-2103.html; "Olle Johansson: Science Experiment at school with Watercress exposed to wifi" http://www.youtube.com/watch?v=WDBAU-F4DW8; *Economic Times* (PTI), 14 June, 2013; http://www.mumbaimirror.com/mumbai/others/Mobiles-to-be-sold-with-safe-use-guides/articleshow/20433035.cms; http://www.telegraph.co.uk/news/worldnews/asia/southkorea/10138403/Surge-in-digital-dementia.html; http://koreajoongangdaily.joins.com/news/article/article.aspx?aid=2973527; Joe Imbriano, *The Fullerton Informer*, 8 May, 2013; http://thewesterlysun.com/news/experts-cellphones-pose-threat-to-children-s-brains/article_cb228b34-e06f-11e2-971b-0019bb2963f4.html; http://ca.finance.yahoo.com/news/ontario-teachers-union-wants-cell-203000914.html; *International Journal of Radiation Biology*, Vol. 84, No. 4, April 2008, pp. 325-335; Citizens for Safe Technology Press Release, 29 July, 2013; http://www.cmaj.ca/content/early/2013/06/24/cmaj.109-4523.full.pdf+html; http://apps.fcc.gov/ecfs/document/view?id=7520941318; John G. West, 'Multifocal Breast Cancer in Young Women with Prolonged Contact between Their Breasts and Their Cellular Phones', *Case Reports in Medicine*, vol. 2013, Article ID 354682, 5 pages, 2013. doi:10.1155/2013/354682; Cindy Sage and Martha Herbert, Chapter 20 *Bioinitiative Report* 2012; http://timesofindia.indiatimes.com/city/kolkata/Study-puts-glare-back-on-cell-tower-risks/articleshow/27492794.cms; Prithvijit Mitra,TNN, Dec 17, 2013; http://www.news.com.au/technology/dr-marietherese-gibson-resigns-from-tangara-school-for-girls-over-wifi-health-worries/story-e6frfrnr-1226729172333#ixzz2gOOUTvdv; Eileen O'Connor report on SCENIHR, Athens, 27-28 March, 2014; http://betweenrockandhardplace.

wordpress.com/2014/10/18/former-nokia-technology-chief-mobile-phones-wrecked-my-health/; http://www.timeslive.co.za/thetimes/2014/12/11/cellphones-fry-young-brains; http://onforb.es/1u3sYMd.

4: Britons Enslav'd?

Interview with Michael Bevington, 18 February, 2013.

5: Doctor, Doctor

Interviews with Dr Erica Mallery-Blythe; Dr Andrew Tresidder; Dr Diana Samways; The Undercover Epidemiologist.

6: The Scientific Silence (Why Microwaves Cause Cancer in Canada, Russia, China, America and India, and Are 'Safe' in the UK)

Interviews with Brian Stein; Alasdair Philips correspondence; Professor Andrew Goldsworthy various correspondence.

7: Free Russia (Why the Former Communist World Leads the Way)

'Overview of Health Effects of Extremely Low Frequency Electromagnetic Fields', N. Rubtsova, RAMS Institute of Occupational Health, Moscow, Russian Federation; 'Hygienic, clinical and epidemiological analysis of disturbances induced by radio frequency EMF exposure in human body', V.N Nikitina, North-West Scientific Centre of Hygiene and Public Health, St Petersburg, Russia, 16-17 October, 2000; Professor Yury Grigoriev, EMF Workshop Brussels, 20 February, 2013; RRT Press Release; ITAR-TASS News Agency, Moscow, 11 March, 2014; Professor Oleg Gigoriev, EMF Workshop, London, 13 June, 2015.

8: Following the Money

Alasdair Philips correspondence; interview with franchisee; http://deccanherald.com/content/294813/no-mobile-towers-near-schools.html; Sarah Dacre, *Lifescape* magazine, April 2007; Sarah Knapton, *Daily Telegraph*, 30 March 2017; http://timesofindia.indiatimes.com/city/kolkata/Study-puts-glare-back-on-cell-tower-risks/articleshow/27492794.cms and Prithvijit Mitra,TNN, 17 December, 2013; Site Finder website; www.mastsanity.org; Interview with 'S-J', 2014; Elizabeth Barris correspondence, 2014; Swiss Re SONAR – *Emerging Risk Insights*, http://www.takebackyourpower.net/news/2014/03/31/major-insurance-firm-swiss-re-warns-of-large-losses-from-unforeseen-consequences-of-wireless-technologies/; *Bermuda: Re+ILS*, 12 April, 2013; http://www.businesswire.com/news/home/20150511005200/en/International-Scientists-Appeal-U.N.-Protect-Humans-Wildlife-#.VVDe5PCoiQU; Subject: EMF ALLIANCE INTERNATIONAL: 20 Organisations Complain to the European Commission about the SCENIHR 2015 Opinion - Wed, 9 Sept 2015 2:55 PM: Jenny Fry various coverage in the *Independent*, *Daily Mirror* and *Daily Telegraph*, 1 December 2015: Debra Fry email to Phillip Watts, 1 May, 2016: NTP study coverage in *Microwave News* May 2016 and various: The *Times*, 8 November, 2018; Minutes of New Hampshire and Oregon legislative assembly bills, *The Microwave Factor*, 25 July, 2019; EM-Radiation Research Trust 'Radiation Health 2019: Get the Facts' Conference, London, 28 September, 2019: FeganScott, San Francisco, 9 December 2019: PhonegateAlert website, January 2020: *Financial Times*, 15 February, 2020: EM-Radiation Research Trust and Environmental Health Trust coverage 2019 and 2020.

9: The Birds and the Bees (and the Rats and the Bats)

Dr Ulrich Warnke, 'Bees, Birds and People: The Destruction of Nature as a result of 'Electrosmog'; The Human Ecological Social Economic project, UK; www.hese-project.org/en/; Ritz T et al. 'Resonance effects indicate a radical-pair mechanism for avian magnetic compass', *Nature* 2004, May 13, Vol 429, p. 177; Geoffrey Lean, *Independent*, 7 September 2008; Kompetenzinitiative bulletin, Berlin, 16 March, 2008; http://www.newscientist.com/article/dn23203-flowers-get-an-electrifying-buzz-out-of-visiting-bees.html; http://www.sciencemag.org/content/early/2013/02/20/science.1230883; Johansson and Goldsworthy correspondence; Bat Conservation Trust; www.bats.org.uk; Ministry of Environment and Forests, Government of India; moef.nic.in; http://www.ncbi.nlm.nih.gov/pubmed/20560769; Electromagn Biol Med. 2010 Jun;29(1-2):31-5. doi: 10.3109/15368371003685363.

10: One of Us

Interviews with Brian Stein, 2012-2020; Brian Stein diaries 2005-2020; *'For a good night's sleep, stop taking the tablets'*: The Times, 17.11.2015; *'Smartphones Make Us Dumb'* :The Times, 11.10.2015; The Times, 12.10.2015; The Times, 11.11.2015; Happiness Institute in Copenhagen; The Times, 15.10.2015; The Times, 17.11.2015; The Times 5.2.2018; The Daily Mail, 21.6.2018.

GLOSSARY OF TERMS

1G: First generation wireless roll-out.

2G: Second generation wireless roll-out.

3G: Third generation wireless roll-out.

4G: Fourth generation wireless roll-out.

5G: Fifth generation wireless roll-out.

Bandwidth: The range of frequencies available via government auction to mobile phone suppliers.

Base station: A fixed transceiver connecting mobile devices to networks.

DECT: Digitally Enabled Cordless Telephone.

ES: Electrically Sensitive.

EHS: Electrically Hypersensitive.

ELF: Extremely Low Frequency.

EMF: Electromagnetic Field.

Electrosmog: The term coined for the prevalence of electromagnetic fields, increasingly of a man-made, wireless, high frequency, non-ionising radiation nature, in everyday life.

Epidemiology: The study of the determinance and prevalence of diseases in populations.

Frequency: The number of oscillations per second measured in hertz (Hz). In the field of wireless communication, kilohertz = 1,000 HZ, megahertz = 1,000,000 Hz, gigahertz = 1,000,000,000 Hz.

GSM: Global System for Mobile Communications.

High-frequency radiation: Non-ionising radiation with a frequency of 30 kilohertz to 300 gigahertz. Mobile telephony and wireless communications use this property for wireless data transmission.

ICNIRP: International Commission on Non-Ionising Radiation Protection, the regulatory body closely associated with the mobile 'phone industry and scientists and psychologists employed by them.

Ionising radiation: Electromagnetic radiation that has enough energy to ionise or break chemical bonds – for example, X-Rays.

Non-Ionising radiation: Electromagnetic radiation that was once thought unable to carry enough energy to ionise or break atoms, molecules or chemical bonds and alter the bioactivity of living organisms: for example, microwaves. Independent peer-reviewed scientific research shows that it can and does.

RFR: Radio Frequency Radiation.

SAR: Specific Absorption rate. The level of energy emitted by a mobile device set by mobile phone manufacturers and the wireless industry deemed to be safe for the user. Industry-funded and independent scientists disagree over the definition between thermal and non-thermal effects, scope and validity of current safety levels.

TETRA mast: Terrestrial trunked radio masts used by government and services such as police and army.

'War-Gaming': The mobile phone industry term for replicating independent scientific research in order to discredit it.

White Zone: An area free from microwave radiation.

Wi-Fi: The term first coined by Interbrand in 1999 and a play on 'Hi-Fi'.

WLAN: Wireless Local Area Network.

USEFUL WEBSITES FOR RESEARCH, INFORMATION AND ADVICE

The Microwave Factor emfrefugee.blogspot.com is the definitive international resource for research, information and advice on the hazards to public health from microwave radiation and 5G.

Radiation Research Trust www.radiationresearchtrust.org is the leading UK resource for research, information and advice.

Microwave News https://microwavenews.com founded and led by Dr. Louis Slesin in the USA is an authoritative independent media source of information about the mobile phone industry, industry tactics over the past decades and the history of independent scientific research showing the inadequacy of mobile phone operators' safety standards.

Environmental Health Trust ehtrust.org Led by Dr. Devra Davis, EHT based in the USA is a leading resource in the campaign for a safer mobile and Wi-Fi industry worldwide.

USEFUL PUBLICATIONS

Birds, Bees and People: The Destruction of Nature by Electrosmog Ulrich Warnke

Black on White – about Electrohypersensitivity Rigmor Granlund-Lind, John Lind, Sweden 2005.

Cell Phones: Invisible Hazards in the Wireless Age George Carlo and Martin Schram

Crosscurrents Robert Becker

Digital Dementia Dr Manfred Spitzer

Dirty Electricity: Electrification and the Diseases of Civilisation Samuel Milham, 2010

Disconnect: What the Cell 'Phone Industry Doesn't Want You to Know About Radiation Concerns Devra Davis

EHS and a Novel Neurological Condition Andrew Marino, 2011

The EHS Workbook: A Guided Journey to Feeling Better Angela Hobbs

EMF Information for Schools Dr Elizabeth Evans MA, MBBBS, DRCOG

Electromagnetic Sensitivity and Electromagnetic Hypersensitivity: A Summary Michael Bevington

The Force: Living Safely in a World of Electromagnetic Pollution Lyn McLean

Going Nowhere Andrew Marino and D. McCarty

How to Beat Electrical Sensitivity Lloyd Burrell

Ill Health From Wi-Fi ES-UK Information Sheet 11

I'm a Patient... Get Me Out of Here Dr Diana Samways

Mobile Communications and Public Health edited by Marko Markov with contributions from Professor Yury Grigoriev. Published in Britain by Taylor and Francis. The book is also distributed in the US.

Resonance James Russell

The Body Electric Robert Becker

Wireless Smart Meters and People with ElectroSensitivity ES-UK Information Sheet 14

ACKNOWLEDGEMENTS

In North America:

Elizabeth Barris, Dr Martin Blank, George Carlo, David Carpinter M.D, Frank Clegg, Dr Devra Davis, Environmental Health Trust, Andre Fauteux, Dr Magda Havas, Elizabeth Kelley, Dr Henry Lai, Dr. B. Blake Levitt, Dr Andrew Marino, Dr Samuel Milham, Dr Ron Melnick, Lloyd Mogan, Dr Joel Moskowitz, Janet Newton, Barb Payne, Professor Martin Pell, Camilla Rees, Cindy Sage, Dr Louis Slesin.

In Europe and the UK:

Mike Bell, Professor Fiorella Belpoggi, Michael Bevington, Lloyd Burrell, Mark Crispin Miller, ES-UK, Dr Elizabeth Evans, Dr Ian Gibson, Professor Andrew Goldsworthy, Professor Oleg Grigoriev, Professor Yury Grigoriev, Sissell Halmoy, Professor Lennart Hardell, Professor Denis Henshaw, *Investigate Europe*, Professor Olle Johansson, Kompetenzinitiative, Professor Michael Kundi, Professor Dariusz Leszczynski, Dr Erica Mallery-Blythe, Mike Mitcham, Dr Gerd Oberfeld, Eileen O'Connor, Dr Peter Ohnsorge, Dr Dimitris Papagopoulos, Alasdair Philips, Graham Philips, Jessica Purkiss, Radiation Research Trust, Alison Rudkin, James Russell, Dr Diana Samways, Anne Silk, Dr Sarah Starkey, Antoinette Stein, Sir William Stewart, Dr Andrew Tresidder, the Undercover Epidemiologist, Dr Andrea Vornoli, Professor Ulrich Warnke.

In Australia:

Dr Don Maish.

And others who prefer to remain anonymous.

APPENDICES 1-9

The appendices referred to in the text are among the leading independent scientific studies of the effects of non-thermal microwave radiation on human and animal health and living organisms.

These and many more studies are available to read or download for free from the EM-Radiation Research Trust website * www.radiationresearch.org and other links listed below.

The papers presented by speakers at 'Radiation Health 2019: Get the Facts' are also available on the website with news and updates concerning the latest developments in the campaign to call the mobile phone industry to account and make Wi-Fi safer around the world.

Appendix 1: List of Independent Studies of the Effects of Microwave Radiation

http://www.es-uk.info/wp-content/uploads/2018/05/Selected%20ES%20and%20EHS%20studies.pdf

www.radiationresearch.org

Appendix 2: Professor Andrew Goldsworthy Study

'The direct electrical effect on our cells, organs and tissues does far more damage to us at energy levels that may be hundreds or thousands of times lower than those that cause significant heating. These are termed non-thermal effects. As yet our governments and health authorities are doing nothing to protect us from them.'

www.radiationresearch.org

Appendix 3: Michael Carlberg and Lennart Hardell Study

'On the association between glioma, wireless phones, heredity and ionising radiation' Michael Carlberg, Lennart Hardell

Department of Oncology, University Hospital, SE-701 85 Örebro, Sweden Accepted 6 July 2012

'Certainly results from the Hardell group as well from the Interphone group show an increased risk for glioma associated with long-term mobile phone use. Also use of cordless phones increases the risk when properly assessed and analysed. The risk is highest for ipsilateral exposure to the brain of RF-EMF emissions. Adolescents seem to be at higher risk than adults.'

www.radiationresearch.org

Appendix 4: B. Blake Levitt and Dr Henry Lai Study

'Electromagnetic radiation emitted by cell tower base stations and other antenna arrays'

'The increasing popularity of wireless technologies makes understanding actual environmental exposures more critical with each passing day. This also includes any potential effects on wildlife.'

www.radiationresearch.org

Appendix 5: T-Mobil/Ecolog Study

'A lowering of the guidelines to a maximum of 0.5 W/m^2 should urgently be considered.'

'A particular problem in this exposure group is posed by children and adolescents, not only because their organism is still developing and therefore particularly susceptible, but also because many adolescents have come to be the most regular users of mobile phones.'

'Advertising towards this population group should be banned.'

www.radiationresearch.org

Appendix 6: Sarah Starkey Report on Vested Interests between ICNIRP and AGNIR

'Public health and the wellbeing of other species in the natural world cannot be protected when evidence of harm, no matter how inconvenient, is covered up.'

www.radiationresearch.org

Appendix 7: National Toxicology Program Study and Peer Review

https://ehtrust.org

Download the NIEHS/NTP Peer Review Report

Download NIEHS/NTP issued PDF of Peer Reviewers Conclusions

Download Presentation by Dr. Michael Wyde NTP Summarizing the NTP

www.radiationresearch.org

Appendix 8: Ramazzini Institute Study

https://ehtrust.org

Ramazzini Study On Radiofrequency Cell Phone Radiation: The World's Largest Animal Study On Cell Tower Radiation Confirms Cancer Link

www.radiationresearch.org

Appendix 9: The European Parliament Report 'The International Commission on Non-Ionizing Radiation Protection (ICNIRP): Conflicts of interest, corporate interests and the push for 5G.'

'That is the most important conclusion of this report: for really independent scientific advice we cannot rely on ICNIRP.'

For the full text of this report see EM-Radiation Research Trust and Environmental Health Trust (EHT) websites.

www.radiationresearch.org

https://ehtrust.org

THE AUTHORS

Brian Stein CBE is a successful retired business leader and chairman of the EM-Radiation Research Trust.

Jonathan Mantle's books are published in 30 countries and 16 languages. He is not as far as he knows electrically sensitive.